HEAL ENDOMETRIOSIS NATURALLY

Heal Endometriosis Naturally - WITHOUT Painkillers, Drugs or Surgery

Wendy K Laidlaw

ISBN-10: 1515385698
ISBN-13: 978-1515385691

DEDICATION

I dedicate this book to my two beautiful and wonderful children, Maxine and Sebastian.

Several medical professionals told me many times that I would never have children; so you both are a testament for others – so they may know it is important to *never* give up hope.

You are both are my light, my bright joy, and my inspiration in the world. I am so incredibly proud you both for the resourceful, passionate and delightful young people you have become.

I love you both more than I could ever put into words, and I thank God every day being lucky enough to have you both as my children and in my life.

All my love always,

Mummy xx

MEDICAL DISCLAIMER

THIS BOOK IS BASED ON MY PERSONAL EXPERIENCES ONLY, AND SHOULD NOT BE USED TO TAKE THE PLACE OF A MEDICAL PROFESSIONAL'S OPINION.

I am not a scientist nor am I a medical expert on endometriosis. I am a woman's health coach and consultant, who had previously suffered from endometriosis and has read and studied a great deal about the subject. During my recovery I retrained in nutritional therapy, psychotherapy and psychology which is ongoing, but by no means, have I studied this subject of endometriosis completely and exhaustively.

What I bring to the book is over 33 years worth of my own healing journey, my experiences and processes that led to my full recovery from the pelvic pain and symptoms of endometriosis and adenomyosis. What I describe is a multi-dimensional, pragmatic approach and principles to healing and recovering using naturally methods which worked well for me and changed my life.

I am unable to make any claims for legal purposes and cannot promise the principles in this book will work for everyone; I can only state what worked for me. Although these principles may not work for everyone, I dearly hope and pray that they work for you, as they did for me, so you can be free of this chronic debilitating condition as well.

The information should not be treated as a substitute for professional medical advice. What is contained within the book is only my experience.

- This book is not intended to replace the medical advice of physicians or doctors. However, I would suggest you seek a medical professional who is supportive of your desire to consider a natural approach to healing. The reader should regularly consult a physician or doctor in matters relating to her health and particularly, with respect to any symptoms that may require diagnosis and/or medical attention.

■ If you think you may be suffering from any medical condition, worsening of symptoms or any new symptoms that are not resolving, you should seek immediate medical attention, and insist symptoms are investigated by tests that are beyond the scope of this book.

Please feel free to ask your doctor or physician to contact me to discuss any aspect of advice suggested in the book. If you have any specific questions about any medical matter you should consult your doctor or other professional healthcare providers.

Please use this book responsibly. You should *never* delay seeking medical advice, disregard medical advice, or discontinue medical treatment because of the information presented in this book.

Readers are advised to take full responsibility for their own safety and know their limits. The author does not take any responsibility for anybody who misuses the advice in the book.

CONTENTS

ACKNOWLEDGMENTS

There are so many people I want to thank for being willing to share their ideas with me. Ideas that ultimately became the strategies and principles behind everything inside of this book.

While there are hundreds of people I have learned from, there are many people who gave me specific ideas for this book. I've tried to give credit to original sources when possible but some of these people may be left out. So I want to mention a few of the brilliant men and women who have inspired me in no particular order.

There are three wonderful, 'wise women' who I want to thank for they are all pioneers in their own field. These women have challenged the conventional 'medical machine' and taken the road less travelled in their passionate attempts to help their patients and clients; Dian Shepperson Mills in nutritional therapy and her book 'Endometriosis: A Guide to Healing Through Nutrition', Nora Covey in the preservation of the womb through her charity Hysterectomy Education Resources and Services (HERS) and her book 'The 'H' Word', and Dr Sarah Myhill in recovering from chronic fatigue syndrome. Thank you to you all for your unwavering faith in me, delightful strength of character, and for holding the torch to lead the way for my recovery through many dark times.

I also want to thank Suzy Grieve who first introduced me to the concept of life coaching and another way of living my life through her The Big Leap programme, Jess Thompson from The Optimum Health Clinic in London, Lion Goodman through his wonderful The Belief Closet programme, Dr Tony Coope for his kindness and patience, and Julia Cameron through her book 'The Artist Way'. They have all been instrumental in my recovery and I thank them for their patience and kindness when I felt lost.

Last, but my no means least, I want to thank Pam Williamson for her professionalism, reliability, consistency and patience as she guided me through some very turbulent times. Her support and belief in me has given me the ability to write this book and make this process available to other women.

Introduction

* * *

The definition of insanity is doing the same thing over and over and expecting different results - Albert Einstein

The pain of endometriosis is a unique and chronic experience. The pain can be dragging, scraping, and pulling. It will often feel like barbed wire rubbing up and down your insides. The occurrence of pain happens every few weeks or days and sometimes, the pain doesn't lessen at all during an endometriosis experience.

You go to your doctor but many doctors will not understand the condition right away, if they ever at all. Some will make you feel that you are making it up. Some might insinuate that you are somehow imagining it and you are 'neurotic'. Some will give you birth control pills and painkillers, but, the pain still lingers.

You may feel depressed, lost, and alone. You just want to get on and live your life but you're tired. Your body is weakened by the constant pain and the disease may drag you down.

You may have thought that once you had a diagnosis that all would become better for you. You may even have had surgery to get a diagnosis and you had hoped that the surgery would be the cure. You may have got worse after the surgery and then, sought another, then another. However, surgeries can cause adhesions, like the white skin on top of a chicken breast, which then attaches itself to other organs and pulls and drags them or ties them in knots; which is yet another complication and side effect to add into the mix of many others.

Millions of women, who have endometriosis, know how utterly debilitating it is. The unexpected nature of this invisible disease makes it difficult to prepare or plan ahead from one month to the next. The pain can make you double up in an instant or send you to bed for two to three days on end. You try to explain the wide varying array of pain to friends, family or work colleagues but they will never understand unless they have endometriosis themselves. How can they? On the outside, you 'look okay' even if your insides are screaming in agony. Having endometriosis can really cause you to feel lonely. You just put up with the pain and hug the hot water bottle tighter, it becoming your closest friend.

Ten years ago, estimates showed that one in every twenty women suffered from Endometriosis. In 2015, figures estimate a terrifying one in every six suffer from it - let's look at it this way - that is about 200 million women worldwide. Now, that is a lot of women suffering needlessly. The invention of social mediums on the internet such as health forums, Twitter, and Facebook have allowed more women to come together to share their pain and despair. We are not as alone as we thought we were.

What really concerns me, as someone who suffered extensively for 33 years, is the lack of information about the alternative options available to women. The medical profession relies heavily on the pharmaceutical and surgical routes when they process women with this disease, but they do not address the underlying causes. Doctors prescribe women full of chemicals or cut them open in surgery and damage them for life. Very few medical practitioners ever fully explain the real horrors and long-term side effects of the 'gold standard' procedures offered to women.

The emergence of charities like Hysterectomy Education Resources and Services (HERS) and The She Trust saved me from a lot of heartache and the information they provided allowed me to retain my uterus. Sadly, these organisations are the minority and a lot more needs to be done in the front end to educate all women, especially young girls, upon the commencement of menstruation that period pains are not 'normal'. Young girls need to learn how to empower themselves to heal before endometriosis becomes a problem. Prevention is far better than a cure.

This book will explore some of the causes of endometriosis. I believe the compounding effect of dioxins, toxins, plastics, parabens, genetically modified foods, pesticides, chemicals, poor diet, and poor nutrition combined can cause severe hormone imbalances. Our impatient society with the 'better, faster, more, now' pressure, add together to activate, increase stress and intensify the pain that is uniquely endometriosis. I will also explain the genetic component, which is widely believed by the medical profession as the major cause of endometriosis.

We will dispel the beliefs, "there is no other option", "I have to take pharmaceutical drugs", "I have to get a surgical diagnosis" and "I have to have another operation", that holds many women stuck in the 'Medical Machine' and back from taking the power they have into their own hands. We will help demystify the healing process by explaining how the body works and how even a small change can make a big difference. It tackles your self-doubts, concerns, and worries about time, money, and feeling alone.

This is a step-by-step approach that enables you to understand and do all of the following:

* Start on your own path to healing by learning how to heal endometriosis naturally

* Break the barriers that are preventing you from owning your own power

* Learn that it is *never* too late to walk away from the medical machine

* Then use your new knowledge to help other women with endometriosis out of pain

We are all aware of how DNA and genetics become some of the main factors for a person to have a disease or condition, however, external and environmental factors are mostly the triggers that develop it. We often ask why only one in a family of four sisters develops the condition and not the others. What are the predisposing factors that affect some women and make them more at risk of developing the condition? These questions are some that I will be tackling in this book.

Endometriosis is an estrogen dominant condition believed to be caused and triggered by a combination of different aspects which will be explained. This book tries to address those different aspects through a multi layer approach and principles. Like peeling back the layers of an onion, you will be uncovering and attempting to identify what the triggers are. Once identified, then, the book will show you how to eliminate and swap them out with natural alternatives. Where many alternative therapies fail is by falling into the trap of claiming a symptom is a single cause that affects everyone. However, Heal Endometriosis Naturally is an integrative approach taking a holistic view of the whole person.

The principle behind this book is to gently, but slowly and consistently, guide you out of the medical machine and the maze of pharmaceuticals, drugs and surgery. Then to introduce you to the wonder that is your body: the body that is ALWAYS wanting to heal itself - so that ultimately, you will have a pain free body.

The book will also look at my journey of suffering and recovery. How I found, after three decades of endometriosis that prevented me from planning - or living - a normal life, a natural way out that healed my endometriosis pelvic appendicitis-like pain, the heavy flows, the clots, the cramps, the bloating, and suffering I experienced. I will explain how I achieved this without the involvement of any medical practices or drugs.

I reached my symptom-free goal with my uterus intact through understanding the premise that the body always wants to heal itself and that has to be our starting position. Then I learned how to peel back, slowly, the layers of my body, my brain and my life to uncover what, why, how - and who, was causing me the pain and stopping me from healing.

It was not an easy journey, but it has changed my life. I am far better today than I have ever been.

I look forward to you joining me.

Now, let's begin…

You are now on a journey, on the right path, with a roadmap in hand, to healing yourself naturally.

Wendy K Laidlaw

Chapter 1 -

A Woman with Endometriosis - Why Me?

* * *

We are what we repeatedly do. Excellence, then, is not an act, but a habit - Aristotle

I could barely pronounce its name when I first

became aware of endometriosis (which is pronounced as En-doe-mee-tree-O-sis), but I certainly knew its symptoms. I had my first monthly cycle at age 11 and it was awful. Unlike all my school friends, I was in endless pain every month since the beginning. Back then, I felt like I was the only one who suffered terribly. None of my friends seemed to be as troubled as I was or have the chronic cramps I had. Their periods would come and go without a hitch. From that point on, I strived hard to ignore the pain; I even used the 'mind over matter', positive thinking mindset to try and will the pain away, and pretend all was okay every month.

For the next 30 years, I would come to dread every arrival of my menstrual cycle. The initiation into adulthood was so embarrassing with the crippling period pains, which ensued without abatement month in, month out, year after year. Barbed wire scraping, acute appendicitis-like throbbing, beating, pounding, pulsing, flashing, shooting, jumping, sharp, cutting, lacerating, gnawing, wrenching, pulling, searing, tingling, sickening, suffocating, gruelling, agonising, torturing, and piercing are just some of the words that can be used to describe the pain. It was like an endless endurance test. An endurance test that I felt I was losing every month. I came to dread anyone asking me how I was. I would pretend and say "I'm fine" for I feared telling them the truth would sound like I was feeling sorry for myself.

The dragging sensations in my pelvis would travel down my legs, around my lower back and the headaches would turn into migraines. I was always tired, exhausted and out of energy. I kept myself going by pumping up on sugar, which I grazed on all day. That was the only way I could function properly, and I needed it especially when I had a full time business, family and house to run by the time I reached 40 years old.

I would always experience a heavy flow and flooding of dark red thick blood clots every period. Oh, the flooding scared me when I was young – I always thought I was dying. I used to wonder how you could lose so much blood in a day and still live. It would literally pour out of me leaving me drained, weak and utterly exhausted. Not surprisingly the heavy flow caused me to have an aversion to wearing white or light coloured trousers. The sanitary pads in the 1970s and even some of the modern ones today, could not contain my flow. I usually ended up either staying indoors or as close to a toilet as possible, at all times, during the first 3-4 days of my period.

I was officially diagnosed with severe stage IV endometriosis at fifteen years old. The pain had become so unbearable that my mother had to make an appointment with a gynaecologist. That appointment at the gynaecologist's office still lives in my memory today as if it was just yesterday. The unpleasant procedure of a stranger doing an 'internal' examination and roughly feeling the inside of my body, as I lay there frozen to the spot dressed in my school uniform with the consultant and my mother looking down on; it was so humiliating. Although I received an official diagnosis of endometriosis that day I was given no explanation of why, what or how it had taken up residence in my body. The gynaecologist merely said it was hereditary, that I was unlucky, and told me that pregnancy would cure it or that I needed to go on the birth control pill.

Well, the gynaecologist was right about one thing, the condition I had was indeed hereditary. My mother had an extreme and severe case of endometriosis too when she was young. She told me stories about how the doctors would gather around her bed in the hospital after another operation and how they were excited to observe her recovery because the extent of the disease which had become widespread in her abdomen. The doctors back then held firm to their belief and their theory that the condition was genetic. However, my grandmother never suffered from it, nor her three sisters or any other distant female relatives. The doctors also told my mother her condition was so severe that it was unlikely she would ever have children. This would not be the first time she proved the medical professionals wrong, because she went on to give birth to my brother and me.

There is a popular train of thought within the gynaecological profession that pregnancy cures endometriosis. This theory proved incorrect for my mother as she constantly went in and out of hospital with chocolate cysts the size of oranges and countless other cysts. In her 40's, she was 'sold' by the gynaecologist on the idea that a hysterectomy would cure her ailments for good. "No more bleeding and no more pain" he said. They were right about the bleeding, but not about the pain. The hysterectomy operation did take away some of the old symptoms but created many new worse ones. Despite the removal of my mother's womb, she still experienced a lot of pelvic pain due to inflammation of some of her internal organs and no one explained this to her. We found out later on that some of the endometrial tissues had already migrated outside of the womb, long before the hysterectomy, and that was still causing her problems.

These endometriosis tissues have an abnormal ability to migrate and grow somewhere else; hence, the reason why they call endometriosis the 'Wandering Womb' and medicine has not yet discovered the real reason why. After that operation, my mother's views of doctors and consultants changed and she would often say "doctors bury their mistakes" and "don't trust doctors". Her words would play repeatedly in my head in the coming years and taught me to question everything the doctors told me and to do my own research.

Even though doctors and consultants told me many times that I would never have any children, I ultimately proved all of them wrong, as my mother had done. I first had a beautiful baby girl called Maxine, and then nine years later, despite two damaged fallopian tubes and only part of one ovary left, I gave birth to a handsome little baby boy called Sebastian.

As you can see, it is so easy to look to doctors as all knowing and knowledgeable of you and your body. I do believe that every doctor has the best intentions and an innate desire to help people from ill health, but only you know your own body; you know it better than anyone else knows, and never forget that.

There are numerous reasons - such as toxins, stress, work, relationship issues, and poor health - that mean you lose the ability to listen to your body which we will discuss in later chapters.

Chapter 2 -

Endometriosis Pain

* * *

Destiny is not a matter of chance; it is a matter of choice. It is not something to be waited for; but rather something to be achieved
- William Jennings Bryan

Endometriosis is a disease, which is so profound, that it can negatively impact every single aspect of a woman's life; from the ability to control reproductive choices, to the intimate engagement of an enjoyable sex life, to the ability to plan or go about a normal task.

Endometriosis is a painful disorder among women in which the tissue that normally lines the inside of the uterus, known as the endometrium, grows outside of the uterus. This abnormal growth is called an endometrial implant or lesion. This disease commonly involves the ovaries, the bowel or the tissue lining the pelvis. Although it is very rare that endometrial tissue spread beyond the pelvic region, it has been found in other areas of body, as well as in animals and in men.

During a normal menstrual period, the endometrial tissue, which lines the inside of the uterus, thickens, breaks down and bleeds, sheds, and exits the body. Some inflammatory hormones, which are known as prostaglandins can cause cramping and discomfort and this is medically known as dysmenorrhea. High levels of estrogen lead to a production of an excess of prostaglandin which is a chemical messenger that causes the uterine muscles to contract. The more prostaglandin production the more pain a woman experiences.

However, during a menstrual period for a woman with endometriosis, the endometrial tissue that grew outside of the uterus and now sits in the abdomen, still continues to act as it normally should – it thickens, breaks down, sheds and bleeds, – but the displaced tissue has no way to exit the body and becomes trapped.

Endometriosis in the abdomen results into internal bleeding and inflammation which causes pain and cysts to form. The other surrounding tissue can become irritated, which may eventually develop scar tissue and abnormal tissue, called adhesions, that binds other organs together unnecessarily. Endometriosis often causes severe pelvic pain during menstrual period and it is the primary symptom. Although many women I know normally experience cramping, as in my case with endometriosis, I described it as a continual appendicitis-like pain; the type that takes your breath away, makes you cry out or double up. I have also observed that endometriosis pain tends to increase and spread over time.

What do endometrial implants look like?
Endometrial implants vary widely in size, shape, and colour. Over the years, they may diminish in size or disappear, or they may grow. Early implants are usually very small and look like clear pimples. If they continue to grow they may form flat injured areas (lesions), small nodules or cysts called 'endometriomas', which can range from sizes smaller than a pin head to larger than a grapefruit.

The History of Endometriosis

In ancient Greece physicians referred to the displacement of endometrial tissue outside of the uterus as 'a wandering uterus'. The social belief was that the womb was the origin of all diseases of women which should be confined and controlled. The word 'hysteria' is derived from the Greek language and it means womb.

Aristotle (385-322 BC) believed that hysteria was caused by a discontented uterus and excessive emotions in women, which is why he believed women were unfit to be in politics. Women had no independent existence in ancient Greece and were always under the control of her father and then husband. Because of their poor social standing, women's biology was referred to as 'bad' and therefore, they were not factored into his teachings. This may explain society's aversion to discussing 'women's problems' even today.

The ancient Greeks thought the womb 'moved' in situations of insufficient food, exhaustion, and menstrual suppression. Most of the physical and emotional female illnesses during that Classical Period were described as hysteria. The theory of hysteria and myth of the wandering womb still hold true, some 2500 years later, and continue to influence medical practise and doctors today. For example, in ancient Greece it was believed that sex and pregnancy were ultimate cures, and that when a women did not have intercourse her womb became liable to be displaced and dry.

Modern Day

Many general practitioners (GP's) in the UK are given approximately 10 days training as part of the gynaecological learning and medical training. Women with endometriosis may have put up with severe and prolonged pain over many years before they eventually go to visit their doctor. The doctor may be unaware of the debilitating nature of endometriosis and may dismiss the pain and the woman as hysterical or neurotic. Naturally, this compounds the problem for women. Sometimes a doctor may perform a physical and pelvic exam after collecting a symptom report and medical history. The pelvic examination will evaluate the size and position of the ovaries and check for tender masses or nodules behind the cervix.

If the woman's pain is believed by the doctor then she may be offered the birth control pill or intrauterine coil (IUD). Neither of these contraceptive methods are cures and can often create more endometriosis symptoms and side effects. The woman may get referred to have imaging tests carried out. A non-invasive ultra sound is an imaging technique which is performed in cases where other conditions are suspected, such as uterine fibroids, ovarian cysts, or ectopic pregnancy. Ultrasound will miss small cysts or endometrial implants but can pick up cysts larger than 1 cm (about 1/3 inch). Other imaging techniques, such as computed tomography (CT) scanning or magnetic resonance imaging (MRI), may occasionally be used. The issue associated with imaging of endometriosis is the training required to identify it and the cost of the procedure if used as a screening tool.

If the woman is persistent with the doctor then she may be referred to a gynaecologist. The gynaecologist may prescribe stronger hormonal drugs or suggest surgery: both which can have severe and life changing side effects which are rarely explained to women.

Many women with endometriosis are left feeling so understandably desperate to get out of chronic pain, they pass over their bodies, trust and control over to virtual strangers in the hope of getting 'cured'. The medical professional never explains that the treatment is merely trying to help manage symptoms, and never address or help to heal the underlying causes. This leaves the woman in an endless cycle of drugs, surgery, complications, side effects and more pain. It is clear that no woman could ever make up the intensity of pain that is endometriosis.

What is cruel however, is that some people in the medical profession do not believe the intensity of pain described and the woman with endometriosis has to 'fight' to be believed.

Chapter 3 -

Endometriosis Symptoms and Causes

✳ ✳ ✳

Know Thyself - Socrates

Thehe symptoms of endometriosis are many and range in frequency and severity based on a number of factors. Some women with endometriosis have a belief that they can only get a diagnosis of endometriosis from a gynaecologist. Unfortunately to get a diagnosis from a gynaecologist invariably means the woman has to have an operation, which is very damaging to their already 'pained' body. Some women go through the trauma of an operation only to have the gynaecologist say they could find nothing; leaving the woman distraught and confused. However, there are other ways to have endometriosis confirmed and this can be by going through a list of common symptoms and a process of elimination. Make sure you find a doctor who is understanding of the condition and supportive. That is very important. You need to have someone believe you and want to work with you to heal yourself.

Change doctors and practises if need be to find someone who will support you. Ideally the doctor will initially want discount any other issues or illnesses and then support your desire to heal naturally. I will be encouraging you to listen to your body and your instincts throughout the book and to develop confidence in your own knowledge of your body.

This is important if you feel you have not been taken seriously by the medical machine before. Whether you have been believed or not by the medical profession, you know your body better than anyone.

Here is a list of the types of symptoms and signs that may point out whether or not you already have or are about to have endometriosis, although this is, by no means, an exhaustive list:

- **Severe pelvic, lower abdominal pain that seems to get worse every menstruation** – The pain may begin at a day or two before and will extend several days into the menstrual period, and may include significant lower back, vagina, leg, and abdominal pain.

- **Heavy prolonged period bleeding with clots** - Heavy blood flow with thick clots and may extend to 7-10 days.

- **Ovulation pain** - Pain may be noticeable at ovulation, day 12-14, as egg is released from the ovary.

- **Bowel or urinary disorders** – You may experience painful bowel movements or urination, or bladder pressure within your menstrual period. Irritable bowel syndrome, constipation or diarrhoea is common.

- **Painful sexual intercourse** – Pain during and/or after having sex is a common symptom with endometriosis. You may be unable to climax, or have spotting or bleeding after sex.

- **Infertility** – Most often, women who seek treatment for infertility are diagnosed with endometriosis.

- **Other symptoms** – Spotting during your cycle, abnormal pap smear, chronic debilitating fatigue/ chronic fatigue syndrome (CFS), fibromyalgia, premenstrual tension (PMT), allergies, migraines, restless leg syndrome, insomnia, night sweats, hot flushes, breast tenderness, water retention, bloating or nausea that tends to worsen every menstrual period, may also be signs of having endometriosis.

Diagnosis

If you have two or more of the above symptoms and have ruled out any other possible causes with your doctor (i.e., all other blood tests for other conditions have come back clear), then, it is highly probable that endometriosis is the cause.

Medical professionals or GP's invariably prescribe hormonal drugs or refer you to a gynaecological consultant to have the diagnosis of endometriosis validated by surgical means: if they can see it.

However, do not underestimate how both these forms of treatment; drugs and surgery, carry great long term, irreversible risks and side effects that can permanently damage the body. Pharmaceuticals merely try and manage symptoms of endometriosis but do not address the underlying causes of the condition. Therefore the process of elimination from the above checklist and consultation with your doctor should be all you need to believe you have the condition.

Although severe pelvic pain is the primary symptom of endometriosis, it is not always a reliable indicator of the extent of the endometriosis condition. I have met some women with only mild endometriosis but experience extensive pain, while I have met others with advanced endometriosis but experience only little pain. Therefore, it is very important to carefully observe and pay keen attention to everything you experience during your every menstrual period. It would be useful to record in a pain journal, or an iTunes App, your pain scores and symptoms. You will want this information to monitor your progress as we move through the book and start adapting the changes.

Causes

The definitive causes of endometriosis remains in debate and are still not certain, which lead it to be called the 'disease of theories'. No single researcher or medical practitioner has found the exact answer but several theories have been formulated from medical records and other studies. I will explain each of them.

- **Retrograde menstruation** - This is one of the most highly favoured explanations for endometriosis. Here, it is theorised, that during retrograde menstruation, the menstrual blood, containing endometrial cells, flows back up through the fallopian tubes and into the pelvic cavity instead of out of the body. These displaced cells will then stick to the pelvic walls and surfaces of the other pelvic organs, where they will grow and continue to thicken and bleed over the course of each menstrual period. Although most medical practitioners generally accept this as the main culprit for endometriosis, there is still no explanation as to why the displaced tissue flows backwards.

- **Immune system or immunologic dysfunction** - It is also possible that a 'broken' immune system or any problems with it can make the body unable to recognise and eliminate the endometrial tissue that is growing outside the uterus.

- **Embryonic cell growth** - All of the cells lining the pelvic and abdominal cavities come from embryonic cells. Whenever one or more of the small areas of the abdominal lining turn into endometrial tissue, endometriosis can and may develop.

- **Transport of endometrial cells** - Another rare possibility, here the lymphatic system of blood vessels and tissue fluids may transport the endometrial cells to other parts of the body.

- **Genetics** - Another favoured theory states, there is a 70% risk in women and girls of inheriting the disease, if their mothers or female relatives have endometriosis.

- **Environmental factors** - Toxins referred to as xenoestrogens and phytoestrogens have been known to cause cell changes and mutations, which cause immune disorders and allow for implantation of menstrual debris. Some 51 xenoestrogen chemicals have been found to officially disrupt human hormonal balance. Tampons, for example, contain traces of dioxins although they may state 100% natural cotton. Xenoestrogens are found in many aspects of our everyday life via pesticide sprayed food, household products and personal care products.

- **Dioxins** - Dioxins are a by-product of chlorinated products and plastics, and second in line to radioactive waste. In 1993, Rhesus monkeys were exposed, over a period of 10 years, to low levels TCDD (2,3,7,8-Tetrachlorodibenzo-p-dioxin), which is a colourless compound without a distinguishable odour. These monkeys subsequently developed reproductive abnormalities and endometriosis. TCDD is known to be a human carcinogen and human exposure is greater than the monkeys were exposed to in the experiment. Many studies have found women with endometriosis have significant levels of dioxin indicated in their bodies.

- **Implantation through surgical scar** - This can occur rarely but it is also possible. For example, after a surgery such as a hysterectomy or a Cesarean section, endometrial cells may attach to the surgical incision.

Although these theories have become a foundation for diagnosing women to have endometriosis, there are other factors that would increase the risk of getting the disease. One such factor favoured by the medical profession is never giving birth; this is based mainly from the fact that almost none of the women who had children before the 1970s had endometriosis. Although, the increase in environmental pollutions is what I believe to be the main cause, which I will cover in more detail later.

Other factors that have been pointed out include; a long history of pelvic infections, abnormalities in the uterus, severe prolonged stress and any medical condition that prevents the normal passage of menstrual flow out of the body. Endometriosis is known to develop a few years after the onset of menstruation, which was not the case with me. The signs and symptoms of this disease will cease temporarily with pregnancy and sometimes, end with menopause; but not always.

Endometriosis can cause many complications including some listed of the below:

Infertility
The main complication that endometriosis brings is infertility or the difficulty of getting pregnant, or not being able to get pregnant at all. About 30% to 50% of women with endometriosis have difficulty getting pregnant. One reason for this is endometriosis can damage the fallopian tubes or the ovaries, which cause fertility problems.

In order for pregnancy to occur, first, an egg is released from an ovary and it will travel down through the neighbouring fallopian tube. Next, a sperm cell will come along to attempt to fertilise the egg cell. Once it is successful, the fertilised egg will attach itself to the wall of the uterus to begin development. An endometriosis condition may obstruct the passage in the fallopian tube and keep the egg and sperm from uniting. In some cases, the condition also seems to affect fertility in less direct ways, such as cause damage to the sperm or egg cell.

In spite of this, it is estimated that up to 70% of women who have mild to moderate conditions of endometriosis can still conceive and will be able to get pregnant without the help of treatment. Treatment using medication does not guarantee improvement of fertility in women with endometriosis. Surgery to remove the visible patches of the endometriosis implants is sometimes considered but then again, this too will not give a guarantee that you will get pregnant and often the pelvic region develops yet more adhesions. Due to the difficulty of dealing with this disease, doctors often advise women with endometriosis not to delay having children as the condition usually worsens with time.

Ovarian Cysts

The other main complication brought about by endometriosis is ovarian cysts. These start out as small fluid-filled cysts on the ovaries which can occur when the endometriosis tissue grows near the ovaries. They may be colourless, red, or very dark brown. When these endometriomas are filled with thick, old, dark brown blood these ovarian cysts, called endometriomas or 'chocolate cysts', can grow large and become incredibly painful. If the cyst bursts then the contents an spill out or empty all over the abdominal cavity and organs causing excruciating pain.

Adhesions

The inflammatory condition and nature of endometriosis can cause repeated scar tissue to form called adhesions. Adhesions are like thin, white chicken skin material that cause an organ to stick or be pulled together with another organ causing intense pain. For example, attaching together the intestines (bowel) or bladder to the abdominal wall. These dense, web-like structures of scar tissue can cause significant pelvic pain, impairing the quality of life, work and social activities.

There is a common misconception that cysts and adhesions complications can be removed by surgery. However, the surgery causes more trauma to the pelvis, more adhesions, and in a high percentage of women their endometriosis symptoms often reoccur in a matter of weeks after the surgery. This can be very disheartening for a woman with endometriosis to have undergone the trauma of an operation only to discover that it has been unsuccessful. The woman is back to square one with very few options and stuck in the maze of the medical machine.

Chapter 4 -

The Medical Machine

* * *

The greatest pleasure in life is doing what people say you cannot do
- Walter Bagehot

The medical establishments in the Western world

have developed some incredible ways to combat illness and diseases to keep us living for longer. The aim of combat ing illness has led to the growth and increased use of pharmaceutical drugs, which in many aspects has been very successful. We have made some great quantum leaps in our health care and generally reap the rewards. The transplanting of hearts, livers and kidneys, to name a few body parts, to the incredible life saving endeavours of the accident and emergency departments in hospitals. No longer is there a worry of dying in childbirth or succumbing to diseases like smallpox or measles. The discovery and development of antibiotics in particular, has been beneficial to many, although increasingly, governments are aware that their effectiveness is declining from overuse. The population have not only come to expect to take antibiotics for even the common cold but to take them repeatedly. Overuse of antibiotics and drugs can mean the development of immunities, chemical sensitivities, allergies and be damaging to the body's own natural defence systems.

The human body is an amazing machine in itself. Our intestines (bowel), for example, has its own 'good' bacteria that combats any 'bad' bacteria that may enter the body through the mouth and into the digestive track. Excess use of drugs and antibiotics kill off this 'good' bacteria, thereby leaving the body vulnerable to yet more infections. Whilst modern medicine has achieved many great feats, the Western world has become increasingly unwell and the prescription of chemical treatments becoming commonplace. Pharmaceutical giants carry great influence over the medical establishments and governments, and one has to question the overuse of them and what underlying natural treatments were used before their invention.

For some diseases like cancer, some radical approaches are taken from chemotherapy to removal of the affected area or organ. However, conditions like endometriosis are harder to diagnose as women may have an array of symptoms. An inexperienced doctor may carry out blood tests and find no 'abnormal' results and conclude that the women with endometriosis is 'making it up' or neurotic. The woman may be dismissed as imagining or exaggerating the pain and prescribed some or any of the following array of pharmaceuticals: pain killers (or nonsteroidal anti-inflammatory drugs (NSAIDs)), or oral contraceptives, intrauterine device (IUD) like Merina coil, Nuva ring, deposhot, or some other synthetic hormone to manipulate the ability to conceive. However, these hormone manipulators prevent ovulation from occurring so less hormones, like progesterone, are produced continuing the body's hormonal imbalance.

Listed below are some of the current medical treatment options that a woman with endometriosis may be routinely offered when she visits her doctor, physician or gynaecologist. This list is a guide and not exclusive.

Some Medical Treatment Options:
- Tens Machine
- Birth control pill/oral contraceptives
- Merina coil/IUD
- Antidepressants
- Painkillers/nonsteroidal anti-inflammatory drugs (NSAIDs); paracetamol, ibruphofen, dihydrocodeine, codeine
- Postap
- Danzol
- Zolodex
- Oramorph
- Propolis
- Cerezette
- Decapeptyl injections
- Pain blockers
- Womb byopsy
- Morphine patches
- Shrinking cyst on ovary
- Cystectomy
- Abdominal Ablation
- Excision surgery
- Diagnostic Laparoscopy
- Hysterectomy - full removal of uterus and ovaries - instant menopausal - osteoporosis
- Opherectomy - removal of uterus leaving ovaries - slow menopause and subsequent surgery when ovaries die off due to insufficient blood supply

Hormonal Treatments

There are over 40 different types of birth control pills which consist of a variation of synthetic estrogen compound and synthetic progesterone called 'progestin'.

It is important to note, and repeat, that **none** of the drugs or hormonal treatments prescribed will eliminate endometriosis. The aim of current medical treatment is to reduce inflammation and try to manage symptoms. However, this rarely happens, and a lot of women may end up having severe side effects and complications. The idea of hormone treatment, with the use of synthetic hormones, is to trick the pituitary gland in to believing you have reached menopause.

Synthetic Progestogen and Progestins

This is important but can be confusing to a lot of women; these products 'progestogen' and 'progestins' are NOT natural progesterone. Note how similar the chemical synthetic pharmaceutical names are to progesterone which you produce in your body. Some synthetic progestogen hormone drugs prescribed are called noresthisterone, dydrogesterone and medroxyprogesterone.

GnRH Analogues

GnRH analogues is a synthetic gonadotrophin releasing hormone to mimic the 3 gonadotropins that the body are produces; lutenizing hormone, follicle-stimulating hormone and chorionic gonadotropin. Some drugs are; Buserelin, Leuprolelin, Nafarelin, Goserelin and Lupron. All these drugs cause serious side effects and in particular Lupron which has as been known to cause serious long term damage to the body.

Merina Coil/IUD

The Merina coil or levonorgestrel intrauterine system is a small 'T' shaped device inserted into the uterus to provide a slow release of synthetic progestin over a number of years. Side effects are ovarian cysts, pelvic pain, weight gain, irregular bleeding, spotting, mood swings, thin and brittle hair. Pelvic infections are common due to the 'string' that hangs down from the coil. The uterus is normally kept sterile, but the string increases the likelihood of infection. Other side effects are extreme pain and bleeding during intercourse if coil is dislodged.

The birth control pills and/or hormonal drugs often cause serious side effects for women with endometriosis, which can cause yet more distress. For example:

- Facial hair on chin, lip, breasts, inner thighs and abdomen
- Excessive weight gain
- Acne
- Deepening of voice
- Depression
- Cardiovascular problems
- Heart attacks
- Damage the digestive system
- Leg swellings
- Damage to the reproductive system
- Hair thinning and hair loss
- Vomiting
- Nausea
- Bloating
- Spotting
- Headaches and Migraines
- Mood Swings
- Breast Tenderness
- Water retention
- Blood clots
- Dizziness

Some of the side effects are irreversible and in some cases side effects are treated with yet more drugs; which cause more side effects. And so the cycle continues.

I visited numerous doctors and gynaecologists over the years and was offered many of the above painkillers, drugs, and surgical options. However, no one ever discussed any other alternatives with me but promoted one drug or hormonal treatment after the next. By the time I had my second child the medical profession referred to my uterus as if it were a redundant organ that needed removing. It was talked about as if there was no other use for it because I was over the age of 40. One gynaecologist even said "I am not sure it is necessary for you to keep it"; like he was referring to an empty crisp packet. I was outraged that an essential female sex organ could be regarded so dismissively.

What bothered me the most was that many women can be put under pressure to make important decisions about drugs and life changing surgical removal of an important organ when they are in great distress and pain. The woman may also be in a vulnerable position. She might be lying in pain in the hospital bed, full of drugs and painkillers, with no make up on and wearing a thin cotton gown, unable to think clearly. This is not the ideal situation to be making life changing decisions or not be fully informed of the risks. Your uterus is a sacred organ and it is essential for a woman's health that it be retained.

Current treatment of endometriosis through the medical machine are many but the real undisclosed fact is NONE of these common drugs and treatments actually address the root causes or underlying triggers of endometriosis. What I did find interesting through my research was that fifty years ago the pharmaceutical giants were not so prominent. The principles were quite different from today and doctors in the 1960's, in USA and UK, would routinely prescribe natural treatments like bio-identical progesterone cream. This was a particularly effective treatment at reducing symptoms and had no side effects. So why did no doctor offer natural bio-identical progesterone cream to me as an option?

Do's and Don'ts with Doctors and Physicians

Be confident and don't be scared to ask lots of questions when visiting your doctor or physician. Do consider making written notes, or ask to record the meeting on your mobile phone when discussing any aspect relating to drugs or surgery. When you are in incredible pain, taking strong pain killers and/or unable to sleep, you may have a fuzzy head and find it difficult to remember or take in any new information you are being given.

Take a trusted friend or family member with you. Many times I took a friend or family member with me and it made a big difference to how I was treated and how confident I felt in asking questions. In fact, on visiting a gynaecologist for a second time I took my partner. The gynaecologist then went on to prescribe and promote a totally different drug to what he had suggested in my first meeting with him; although I later decided to take neither. The list of side effects to the drugs he was recommending were far too disturbing and disruptive to my already pained body.

When you are fully informed about your body and anything you are going to have put in it, or any trauma carried out to it, you are at an enormous advantage to make the right decisions and be under no illusions. Ideally you will reject the conventional medical route and decide the safer option is to move forward towards healing endometriosis using a more natural approach. The natural approach helps identify the sources of pain and to eliminate them. I hope you have realised that painkillers, drugs and surgery only try to manage the symptoms of endometriosis and neglect to address the underlying causes.

If only I had been informed of this many many years ago…

Chapter 5 -

Is Healing Endometriosis 'Naturally' Really an Option?

∗ ∗ ∗

Two roads diverged in a wood, and I.....I took the one less traveled by, and that has made all the difference - Robert Frost

Endometriosis had caused me issues since my first menstruation but after the birth of my son, it got progressively worse. I made regular visits to the gynaecologist who suggested that I take various oral contraceptives, coils and pharmaceutical drugs. The gynaecologist reassured me they would stop my menstrual cycle and 'may' help me with the pain. However, I had been pregnant for 9 months without a menstrual cycle and my symptoms had worsened. So what had gone wrong? I researched online about the side effects to the prescription drugs he was proposing and they were disturbing, and irreversible in some cases. I decided to see if there was an alternative route. I just kept thinking "there has to be another way!".

In fact, it was Hippocrates (460-370 BC), who is often referred to as the 'father of medicine', who sought out natural explanations for natural phenomena, and taught natural means could be employed to fight disease. Although I do not necessarily recommend it, Hippocrates suggested the rubbing of honey on the vagina and chewing of cloves of garlic as some of the ancient treatments prescribed to 'lure the uterus back to its seat'. This all seemed peculiar to me but I decided to do some more investigating.

My research led me to the website called the Endometriosis Society of America. It stated, "if you cut out wheat from your diet your symptoms will disappear". I could not quite believe what I was reading. Was it that simple? Could the removal of wheat remove the pain? I sat there at the computer with a prescription in my hand. The internet was full of stories and warned there could be many possible side effects to the drug I had been prescribed. However, the only other option at that time was to continue with the pain and hope for some kind of miracle. I was aware something had to change. I could not carry on with the level of pain I was experiencing. However, I was not prepared to swap one set of symptoms with other more disturbing and irreversible ones. Something had to give. Could something so simple like removing wheat from my diet really work? I thought "What the heck, it is worth a try! What is the worst thing that can happen? At least I know excluding a food product has no side effects."

After doing further research, I found out that wheat was genetically grown and then modified in the early 1970s. The head of the wheat was made to contain more seeds. This made the plant top-heavy and the crop would fall over. To solve this problem, a hormone was injected into thicken the stalk. Due to the wheat growing so closely together, a fungus started to appear between the stems. This led to another hormone being added to destroy the fungus. It is possible that these two hormones, when absorbed in excess, upset the hormone profiles of women with endometriosis.

I focused on what was essential for me, and that was getting out of pain. It was suggested that the removal of wheat from my diet might attain that. However, to remove wheat from my diet involved quite a big mental shift for me.

My idea of a healthy diet before was actually totally unhealthy. I lived out of local bakeries, I ate fruit scones for breakfast, grazed on sugar items throughout the day and my idea of a vegetable was iceberg lettuce; which is mainly made of water and has little or no nutritional content. I knew nothing of healthy eating. But, my motivation was to get well, educate myself and take full responsibility for my own body. I did not want to take body-altering drugs with horrible side effects. The definition of insanity is doing the same thing over and over and expecting different results; I had to do something differently.

When I went wheat free in the year 2001, there were no commercially available wheat or gluten free products on the market. Even though I was a novice in the kitchen I learnt how to make all sorts of breads like sweet potato bread and stocked up the cupboards with packets of oatcakes. I always carried emergency packets of oatcakes in my handbag from then on incase I was stuck and had nothing to eat. I used to find the prospect of going out to eat so difficult and then people would look at me as if I was an alien when I said I was wheat intolerant. I dropped the 'intolerance' name and soon changed it to 'allergy', which in time stopped the strange questioning looks. I had the odd quivering bottom lip when I would turn up to a cafe or restaurant to find all the main meals had wheat flour in it and there was nothing but potatoes, rice or fruit for me to eat. Although, nowadays, restaurants and cafes are increasingly more aware and accommodating to our wheat free (including gluten and dairy free) dietary needs. There are even sections of supermarket aisles fully dedicated to carrying wheat free and gluten free products in stock, which I still find exciting to this day!

Therefore, the commitment was made and although it was hard to adjust my eating habits and diet initially, within 10 weeks, I felt a significant reduction in pain at ovulation and menstruation. My periods became a 2 - 3 day affair, rather than the 7 - 10 days, and the blood flow became minimal with absolutely no clots. I was ecstatic! Slowly but surely, as the weeks turned into months, I found I was confidently starting to plan ahead and accommodate my new eating regime.

I returned to the gynaecologist and shared with him the exciting developments, encouraging him to share my experience and success with other women. His response however, was he could not share with his other patients, as 'it was not proven through the National Institute of Clinical Excellence (NICE) guidelines'. The message was loud and clear; the medical establishment would be happy to put me on drugs with life changing, and damaging side effects that would keep me in a hamster wheel of symptoms but would not even consider a dietary change suggestion. I was aghast.

I learnt later about all the money and influence the pharmaceutical companies have; they are the biggest business in the Western world, grossing approximately $300 billion dollars a year in sales. Yes, worth repeating: $300 billion a year in sales. Promoting pharmaceuticals and drugs is BIG business. But what about all the poor trusting women who are not told about the real impact of the side effects and how these drugs do not 'cure' or heal endometriosis. These drugs keep them trapped in a vicious medical machine, in a maze of chemicals that end up causing them lifelong damage and do nothing to address the underlying causes.

My gynaecologist later admitted that he had just spent 10 days in an all-expenses paid seminar in Rome, Italy. Paid for by the pharmaceutical company who developed the drug he had been promoting to me. I also learnt that doctors got £100 per intrauterine device (IUD) or coil inserted. It felt dirty, sordid, and wrong.

Chapter 6 -

You Are What You Eat....

* * *

When the going gets tough, the tough get going
- Joseph P Kennedy

R emoving wheat from my diet, and swapping it out for healthier, fresh alternatives, was for me, the first significant step to pain reduction. Within three weeks my pain score reduced by some 50%. It totally surprised me the difference in my body, as it was so simple, yet a profoundly effective course of action. On one occasion I ate a little wheat and immediately the pain hit hard. It was now obvious to me that excluding wheat not only helped with elimination of my menstrual cycle pain and reduction in bleeding, but also bloating and distention of my stomach. Ovulation and menstruation started to come and go without incident. I started to feel I could make social plans again, play with my children, put the hot water bottle away in the cupboard and stop feeling like a bystander in my life. What a huge difference to the quality of my life wheat removal made. One small change made a BIG difference.

Why Wheat?
Ever since man imported grain from the Egyptians and learned how to bake, bread has always been a large part of our diet. Especially during breakfast meals, our society seems

incomplete without bread. However, studies have shown that too much reliance on bread, specifically those made from grains, can actually cause damage to our health. It is not only bread, but we should be careful not to eat too much of anything that contains ingredients from grains. Why is this so? Grains, gluten, and non-gluten products, contain proteins that are not beneficial to your health because they cause irritation and inflammation in your gut.

There are a lot of other grains but why focus only on wheat? There are three main culprits here – gluten, wheat germ agglutinin (WGA) and opioid peptides – all of these are harmful to your body and all of these are found in wheat. Gluten is a compound protein that comprises 80% of the protein found in wheat. Wheat germ agglutinin is a lectin – a protein that binds specifically with sugars – that can be particularly damaging to your health. Opioid peptides are psychoactive chemicals. Those found in wheat are similar to psychoactive drugs like opium or morphine. Now that is truly bad for your health is it not?

Gluten - Gluten has proven to cause gut inflammation in at least 80% of the world's population. Gliadin, the premier problem-causing gluten protein, is similar in structure to other 'good' proteins found in tissues of organs such as the pancreas or the thyroid. Our antibodies that 'hunt' gliadin can end up attacking these organs instead. This results to autoimmune diseases like hypothyroidism and diabetes. Gluten's inflammatory effect in the gut can cause intestinal cells to die prematurely and those cells will oxidize. This effect causes the gut to leak and a leaky gut can allow bacterial proteins and toxic compounds to get into the bloodstream, leading to autoimmune attacks on our body. A leaky gut cannot digest food properly and nutrients are not absorbed fully, thus leading to nutrient deficiencies.

Wheat Germ Agglutinin (WGA) - WGA also acts like gluten by irritating and causing premature cell death in the gut.

WGA disrupts the mucus membrane in the gut to cause bacterial overgrowth and lead to digestive issues such as ulcers. WGA also ends up circulating in our body and in our brain, where it will cause leptin resistance and effects similar to insulin. These two factors can promote obesity. WGA is also known to cause vitamin D stores to deplete quickly. This leads to vitamin D deficiency, weakening of bones, a weakened immune system and a vulnerability to infectious diseases and bacterial attacks.

Opioid peptides. The opioid peptides found in wheat, which are very similar to opioid peptides found in opium, are known to cause addiction to wheat and withdrawal symptoms occur upon the removal of wheat from the diet. These opioid peptides were also noted to be a promoter of Schizophrenia and Schizophrenics often see their symptoms reduce by a lot when they remove wheat from their diets.

Therefore, when it comes to things that we as humans are not adapted to eat, wheat and its gluten protein are probably at the top of the list. Although we can indulge ourselves in less healthy choices once in a while without negative consequences, but wheat and all other gluten containing grains should be avoided, especially for us who suffer the endometriosis condition.

I remember feeling close to tears once when we were out at a friend's house as I did not know what to eat, because everything seemed to have wheat in it. Even some ice creams, sauces and sausages. Meal times felt stressful.

I had a young family and did not want to spend hours thinking or preparing food. I was not a natural comfortable cook. At times, I felt overwhelmed even at the thought of eating. However, I got into juicing organic vegetables, as I found that it was an easy way to get the quantity of vegetables suggested. I bought some simple cookbooks and tried to adopt an approach to food that perhaps my Great

Grandmother or my Cavewoman ancestors would have had. Keeping it simple, fresh, free range, organic and avoiding processed readymade meals filled with additives was my new philosophy. Soups were easy to make and when I used organic vegetables, even my children commented on how good they tasted. One of my favourite soup recipes involved a bag of frozen peas, a chopped up organic onion, a vegetable stock cube, salt, pepper, all mixed into one litre of water. Bring it all to the boil, blend and 'Voila'! A yummy tasty, inexpensive and quick soup loved by all.

Sugar Free
Another aspect of my diet that needed adjustment was my sugar consumption. As I mentioned previously I had survived my days by being pumped up on sugar and used to graze all day long. Why sugar-free? Well, added sugar, the 'sweet poison' of the modern world, as some experts would say, is the single worst ingredient in the diet. Our body already produces its own sugar and only makes enough for what it needs every day. When we eat foods that contain sugar, we disrupt the sugar balance in our body and this becomes 'added sugar'; this is something unwanted in our system. We should always avoid added sugar as if it is the plague. Here are some disturbing reasons why:

Added sugar, like sucrose and high fructose corn syrup for example, does not contain any essential nutrients, just a whole bunch of calories. This is the reason they are called 'empty' calories. There are no proteins, essential fats, vitamins or minerals whatsoever, just pure energy. Sugar is also bad for your teeth because it provides easily digestible energy for the bad bacteria in your mouth.

Why is sugar so bad and what is it made of? Before sugar is allowed to enter the bloodstream from the digestive tract, it is first broken down into two simple sugars – glucose and fructose.

Glucose is found in all living cells on the planet. If we cannot get it from our diet, our body produces it. Fructose is a different case. Our body does not produce it in any significant amount and there is really no physiological need for it. Another thing with fructose is that our liver is the only organ that can metabolize it. This will not be a serious problem if we only eat a little bit of it a time, like from a fruit, or if we just finished exercising, in which case, the fructose is turned into glycogen and stored in the liver until we need it. Now, what if our liver gets full of glycogen and we keep eating more fructose? This results in overloading our liver and forcing it to turn the fructose into fat. If we keep repeating this consumption of large amounts of sugar, we will make our liver fatty and this will cause all sorts of serious health problems.

Sugar causes 'insulin resistance' that leads to metabolic syndrome and diabetes. Insulin is a very important hormone in our body because it allows blood sugar (glucose) to travel to cells from the bloodstream and instructs the cells to start burning glucose instead of fat. Consuming too much sugar causes metabolic dysfunction that forces the insulin hormone to stop working the way it should. This makes the cells 'resistant' to insulin and will no longer burn glucose, resulting in many diseases like obesity, cardiovascular disease and most especially diabetes.

Cancer is one of the world's leading causes of death. It is characterised by uncontrolled growth and multiplication of cancerous cells. One of the key hormones that regulate this kind of growth is insulin. Once insulin stops working due to our uncontrolled consumption of sugar, we become potential victims to cancer.

Why is it so hard to resist eating sweet food? The reason for this is because sugar can cause a massive dopamine release in our brain, which, in turn, creates an addiction to it. Therefore, it will take a lot of will power to totally discipline ourselves and avoid eating food that contains added sugar. We should always instil in our minds the bad effects of too much sugar in our body. This way we can achieve the one thing that truly works for a healthy living – that is abstinence from sugar.

With all the bad things associated with wheat and sugar being fully explained here, I urge you to be aware of what you buy to eat. There is a lot of conflicting nutritional advice about what to avoid and what to eat, and sometimes it can create confusion and frustration. The bottom line is keep your awareness up and read the ingredients list at all times.

Stone Age Diet

Dr. Sarah Myhill is a doctor based in Wales, UK, whose speciality is to help people heal from Chronic Fatigue Syndrome (CFS). I learned to follow Dr. Sarah Myhill's advice "if we simply want to stay well, we should all move towards eating a 'Stone Age' diet based on protein (meat, fish, eggs), fat and vegetable fibre. Western diets get 70% of their calories from wheat, dairy products, sugar and potato, and it is no surprise that these are the major causes of modern ill health such as cancer, heart disease, diabetes, obesity and degenerative disorders."

The image of a Caveman in Stone Age time chasing and killing his supper and dragging it home appealed to me. I understood that food was supposed to be fresh, pesticide free, additive free or hormone free, and importantly, not processed or packaged in plastic in a factory. That was what I sought for me and my family. The phrase "You are what you eat" rang through my head. If I ate rubbish, I felt like rubbish. When I ate healthily, I could feel the difference.

I started eating fresh and organic fruit and vegetables over the non-organic – you really can taste the difference, and it was worth the minimal difference in cost. I would sometimes juice them if I found it hard to eat the recommended five fruit and vegetables a day, or use a 'macro greens' product (wheat free of course) which I put into a drink for an extra body boost. Choose what works for you and remember that little changes can make a big difference, but avoid chemically sprayed, bland tasting, mainstream vegetables.

I also started eating free range, organic, and grass-fed meat and poultry mostly. The difference in taste was really noticeable. As my taste buds improved I started to feel better within my body. I took full advantage of the brilliant online shopping and delivery services offered by most supermarkets. Sometimes I was too busy to even think about shopping, but buying online made it so easy and efficient.

I stopped using the microwave and started cooking the old-fashioned way. I kept trying to think how my grandmother would have bought food, prepared it and cooked it. I eliminated most plastic products, from polystyrene, sippy cups to food wraps, which I found out can release chemicals that act like the sex hormone estrogen, according to a study in *Environmental Health Perspectives:* 'We've long cautioned consumers to avoid extreme heat and cooling for plastics, to discard scratched and worn plastics and we feel like this [study] validates one of our many concerns. "

I got a food intolerance test done to confirm the wheat intolerance. They are inexpensive and can be done by sending a few pieces of hair off to a laboratory where they advise what foods you may be intolerant or allergic too.

You can visit your doctor in the UK and ask to be tested for wheat and gluten intolerances. I am actually okay with gluten; what caused me the greatest pain was the wheat. For some 83% of women with endometriosis it is wheat that is the biggest problem not gluten. If you find excluding wheat alone does not improve your monthly painful ordeal, then it is worth getting gluten sensitivity checked out.

I was advised to avoid soy or soya products at all costs. I had no knowledge about these things before. In fact, I don't think a lot of people realise how hard soy is on their body. I read once in a magazine how women in Japan had fewer period issues because they ate a lot of soy/soya. However, I then, proceeded to eat a tub full of soya nuts and drink soy milk, which resulted in the heaviest haemorrhaging of blood ever on my next monthly period. I was shocked. Soya is a very estrogenic product and needs to be removed from your diet. Avoid drinking soya milk, which is a popular alternative to cow's milk right now. However, do try coconut milk, or rice milk or even goat's milk (which my son uses well) but not soya.

Hypochlorhydria

I did a home test to check my stomach acid which is a condition called hypochlorhydria (HCL). Having good stomach acid is essential for good health but a lot of painkillers and pharmaceutical drugs can damage the intestinal track creating digestion issues. I suffered a lot of discomfort, felt heavy pressure and burning in my stomach after every meal. My GP put me on tablets to reduce acid thinking the pain was due to excess acid, but unfortunately they made me feel worse. I then had a Gastroscopy procedure, which was a tube inserted down my throat, the thickness of your thumb, to inspect my oesophagus and stomach. That was an awful procedure and could have been prevented with a simple home HCL test. What I thought was heartburn and indigestion due to high stomach acid, was in fact the complete opposite and a symptom of stomach acid deficiency.

When the food in your stomach reaches a pH of about 2-4, the valve at the bottom of the stomach (pyloric sphincter) starts to slowly release the stomach contents into the duodenum. From here, the pH raises up and down as it travels through the intestines and out the other end. If the acid in your stomach is insufficient from the beginning, everything from the stomach to the small intestine to the large intestine, will likely be compromised. Without sufficient stomach acid your body cannot break down the food you ingest, therefore no matter what you eat, if it is not likely to be broken down or absorbed, you will not benefit from its full nutrition. Think of it like this: chewing your food is the first crucial step to perfect digestion and stomach acid is the next most important.

To carry out the Baking Soda Stomach Acid home test:

- Mix 1/4 teaspoon of baking soda in 4-6 ounces of cold water first thing in the morning before eating and drinking anything
- Drink the baking soda solution
- Time how long it takes you to burp. Wait up to five minutes to time.

If your stomach is producing adequate amounts of stomach acid you will likely burp within two to three minutes. Burping after three minutes indicates a low acid level. If you have not burped within five minutes, then, it could be an indicator that you have little or no levels of hydrochloric acid in the stomach.

This test is a good indicator but you may want to do more testing to confirm or try to supplement with Betaine HCL tablets on your next meal. I admit I was a little nervous about trying and supplementing with these tablets. I think the name 'acid' made me feel nervous. Betaine hydrochloride (HCL) comes in capsule form so they bypass the teeth (so they are not affected) and despite my initial concern I responded well and lost the pressure, bagged up, and bloated feeling after meals. I was also able to eat protein more easily, as before, I had found it hard to digest these foods. The Betaine HCL also helped improve my bowel function too.

For the next 9 years I excluded wheat, sugar and made adjustments to my diet (referred to as the Endometriosis Diet) and it worked really well for me. Occasionally, if I ever ate wheat without my knowledge, I would feel immediate abdominal cramps and pain, which would take 2 -3 days to subside.

My periods became far more manageable over time and I had no clots and less bleeding. Things seemed to be going well; I started my own property business and started socialising again. Even though I still suffered from exhaustion and chronic fatigue, it was a total relief to be pain free.

Chapter 7 -

Characteristics of an Endometriosis Woman

* * *

The difference between a successful person and others is not a lack of strength, not a lack of knowledge but rather in a lack of will
- Vince Lombardi

So, how does a woman with endometriosis survive in the real world? What are the characteristics of a woman with endometriosis?

Women with this debilitating condition can and will display some very common behavioural characteristics and personality types. From my observations of myself and others, women with endometriosis are fiercely loyal, stoic, determined, strong, lifelong care-givers, and often high achievers. They invariably have very strong mental constitutions (you need to endure the severity and prolonged nature of endometriosis pain) and often put other people ahead of looking after themselves. They are empathetic to the point of losing themselves; they are also thoughtful and kind. Some hold high responsible positions, which can demand a lot from them both physically and mentally. They prefer to operate from a position of control, perfectionism and sense of order, which is often reflected in their personal life as well. It has been said that women with endometriosis hold their real feelings 'deep down and within'.

47

Despite being unwell and constantly suffering pain, women with endometriosis are still able to draw upon their adrenal glands to push themselves forward in their lives. These drawings of adrenals allow them to have the phenomenal energy at times they need to override the pain and fatigue. Little do they know that the adrenals will over compensate and the continual cortisol (a stress hormone) output will aggravate the endometriosis even further, because it will deny the body of any progesterone that may be available.

A hormonal imbalance can be intensified because the body, on a regular basis, is overusing the natural 'fight or flight' mechanism designed to be used only for emergencies and life-threatening situations. This characteristic, plus environmental pollutants, poor diet, nutritional deficiencies and estrogen dominance, explains why endometriosis women find themselves experiencing chronic fatigue, exhaustion, and further autoimmune conditions. The body of a woman is not designed for the constant pull of this particular steroid pathway. One very severe consequence of this action is the total shutdown of ovarian function, which promotes further estrogen dominance, the real driving force behind endometriosis.

In spite of these looming consequences, women with endometriosis interestingly often choose careers that demand excellence, perfection, competition, long working hours, and huge responsibilities. They often go to great lengths in their work and careers. Their work and care taking of others becomes a 'way out' or distraction, because there is a feeling of no control over the disease. The more out of control we are with our own bodies, the more we can drive ourselves harder at work, resulting in holding high and unrealistic expectations of our own performances.

This is proof why some personality experts call endometriosis the 'running away disease' or the 'wandering womb'. Women with endometriosis run away from nurturing themselves and their femininity. They do this by keeping busy and living a high pressured lifestyle, and focusing more on their families, friends, and work, than themselves.

Many women are brought up in a culture that encourages this 'selfless' behaviour. We can feel guilty sometimes even thinking about putting ourselves ahead of another person. The truth is this façade of superwoman-like mentality and physical strength comes about because we, as women who suffer from endometriosis, may believe ourselves to be weakened by our disease. On a subconscious level our frustration and determination is perhaps our driving force. Sadly, though, this can affect our relationship with our body, making us more resentful of our condition and our inability to put ourselves first. We feel we are alone and lost in this condition. This is what drives us to seek approval, acceptance, recognition and self-worth by excelling in our performance, achievements and capabilities: although this can cause great stress.

The 'Oxygen Mask' metaphor is appropriate for women with endometriosis. On an aeroplane, you will hear a flight attendant say to put on your own oxygen mask first before helping another person. Whilst it might feel counter intuitive, no one can help another if they have run out of oxygen and are unconscious. It is very easy for endometriosis women to be 'out there' and become responsible for others. We can end up as the care-givers, the people pleasers, the helpers, the nurturers, and the workaholics, so that we can unknowingly avoid caring for ourselves.

Although our bodies are designed for short bursts of stress, prolonged periods of stress can be damaging to our health. Equally if a woman is doing a job that has no meaning or purpose, or away from people she feels safe or can trust her stress levels will be activated. When a woman receives no empathy or compassion for her endometriosis pain and suffering, or there is great uncertainty in her life, stress levels will be activated. Living in a 'toxic' environment, for example, living with angry neighbours or next to a noisy polluted road can impact on a woman's health. When the body is stressed cortisol, the stress hormone, is realised into the blood stream which suppresses the immune system. When women are emotionally stressed and isolated there is a greater propensity for disease and illness. Disease in our society reflects the lives, environment and culture we live in.

I was lucky enough to work with Suzy Grieve, who is a life coach, author of the books The Big Leap and The Big Peace, and editor of Psychologies Magazine in the UK. Her teachings and philosophy started to open my mind to a concept she referred to as 'my relationship with my body'. Ultimately, at that point, I did not have one. I had viewed my body as this vessel to carry my head around. A head that was perpetually berating, chastising, critical and wracked with anxiety over everything. Suzy introduced the idea that our body is always trying to communicate with us but that many of us have become disconnected from it. When we ignore our body then it 'screams' out at you in pain. Our busy lifestyles mean we spend less time in nature or walking or even sitting in silence, less time listening or hearing our bodies. Suzy also introduced the notion of asking myself the questions: "Who are you at 'pains' to please?", "Who is 'painful' in your life", and "Who drains energy from you?".

Have you heard the parable about the 'Frog in a Pot'? If a frog in placed in a pot of hot water it jumps out immediately to escape the danger. On the other hand, if that same frog is put into a pot of cold water and then that cold water is warmed up slowly to boiling point over time, the frog just becomes 'boiled' to death. The temperature is so gradual, almost imperceptible, that the frog does not realise it is boiling to death.

This was something that, unwittingly, was happening in my life. I was being 'boiled' alive; although, at that time I was not aware of it.

Chapter 8 -

When the Endometriosis Diet Stopped Working...

* * *

What lies behind us and what lies before us, are tiny matters to what lies within us - Ralph Waldo Emerson

Fast forward 9 years after starting the

Endometriosis Diet and in 2010, I ended up in the accident and emergency department of the local hospital writhing around in excruciating pain. Although the endometriosis dietary changes and the elimination of wheat had made a significant reduction in my pain and menstrual cycles for many years, suddenly it was not enough. Something had gone horribly wrong and I did not know what.

I was 43 years old when the endometriosis flare up occurred. I had been aware of an ever-increasing amount of stress building in my work and personal life, and with that my pelvis was feeling increasingly uncomfortable over a period of 6 months. I was aware of many pressures in my life at that time that I used to say 'vampirized my soul', and made me feel like I was 'walking through treacle' every day. I was so disappointed to be back in hospital. Why had the Endometriosis Diet stopped working?

I was in so much agonising pain that the doctors prescribed me double doses of morphine, in addition to 36 painkillers a day. The pain maintained its throbbing and acidic intensity; nothing the doctors gave me lessened the pain. Every morning for the 15 days I was in hospital, the consultant would waltz into the ward with his or her entourage. The consultant would look at the notes on the clipboard for all of about 3 minutes, look down his or her nose at this 'body in a bed' i.e. me, and then prescribe yet some other painkiller or antibiotic. Whenever I questioned or tried to explain that I recognised the symptoms as a flare up of endometriosis I would be patronised with some remark about how it was not possible I could have endometriosis because, a) I had children and b) I had been on no medications or drugs for nine years. And then the entourage would trot off again…

After a few days, when it became obvious the medications were not working, I secretly stopped taking the painkillers the nurses kept giving me. I would take the tablets, wait until the nurses had gone, and then, I would put them into my handbag. I needed to have a clear head. I needed to think, I needed to figure out what to do. I was scared and the pain was intensifying and not reducing and I was still in hospital after 12 days. The painkillers made no difference to the pain but were starting to cause me unpleasant side effects, like breathing difficulties and eczema. I asked to stop the morphine too, which again did nothing for the pain but made me want to vomit continuously (I later learned that this is a common side effect and anti sickness injections should have been given to me). The nurses, the unsung heroes of hospitals, were wonderfully supportive and actually apologetic of the arrogance of some of the doctors and consultants. One nurse even encouraged me to keep taking the morphine so they would understand how ill I truly was. But I couldn't. The drugs were only adding to the problems my body was experiencing.

Fighting to be Believed

After my head was clear of painkillers and morphine, I insisted on speaking to the head of the gynaecological department. I managed to convince him that something was seriously wrong. That same afternoon, I was wheeled into the operating theatre for a diagnostic laparoscopy. Despite previous X-rays, MRI scans, abdominal scans and trans-vaginal scans showing no signs of cysts, endometriosis or adhesions, the laparoscopy confirmed evidence of them all. Prior to this confirmation the doctors had been saying they could see nothing so therefore there must be nothing. This is a common problem for women with endometriosis. They have chronic debilitating pain, but there is no blood test to confirm the condition. Scans or X-rays do not show anything. So instead of the medical profession believing the woman's pain, she is left feeling that she is somehow a hypochondriac and 'making it up'. This belief still continues in the minds of some professionals even now. It is bad enough for women to suffer at all, but then to have to fight to be believed can destroy the soul.

Sadly, I woke up from my surgery still in pain. The nurses shared with me that the notes on my file stated they had found 8 chocolate cysts and endometrial blood fluid in my pelvis. This 'spillage' was the cause of the pain. The hot burning blood from one cyst had burst and emptied its contents all over my uterus, ovaries, bowel and bladder. No wonder I was in so much pain. However temporarily satisfying it was to get confirmation that I wasn't going mad, I soon realised that they had just opened me up but done nothing! The surgeon had opened me up and sewn me back up WITHOUT actually removing any of the offending cysts or liquid. I was distraught - and still in chronic pain.

I was told I would need to be referred to another consultant and get another operation. I was discharged later that day with nothing more than painkillers. I was told I would have to wait 12 weeks on the National Health Service (NHS) to be seen by a consultant gynaecologist. What was I to do in the meantime? No one had any answers. I was just expected to 'put up and shut up'.

My children were very distressed to see me in such pain when I got home. My son and daughter cried when they saw me almost passing out in pain on the bathroom floor over the next few days. My husband worked away from home so I was fully responsible for my children and on my own. I had no one to call upon. I tried very hard to put on a 'brave' face for the children's sake, but it was hard when the pain would come and grab you from nowhere and take your breath away. Or worse, it having you unexpectedly scream out and doubled up in pain.

My local doctor suggested going privately to speed up the process if I could afford it. On the NHS the waiting list was 12 weeks to see the consultant and then a further 9 weeks to have the operation. A total of 21 weeks (about four months) before I might be released from this pain. However, when I went privately, I was able to see the consultant and have the operation within three days!

It cost me several thousand pounds of my savings, but the following week I had a radical abdominal excision and cystectomy to remove all endometrial deposits, cysts and adhesions. I viewed it like I was a car going in for its 10 year service. I thought I was going to be wheeled in, cut open, 'cleaned out', sewn back up and be back up on my feet, like new, within a few weeks.

Then I Got Worse and Worse...

Six weeks after the private operation, and although the acid pain had gone, I had started to develop new disturbing symptoms and pain. I was troubled with a new deep, throbbing, contraction-like pain and pressure in my lower abdomen. I emailed the consultant and he reassured me to 'give it time' as it was probably the body still healing. After 10 weeks, I felt no better. I was starting to get distraught. I was getting worse and worse, not better. This new pain kept intensifying and felt like I was about to give birth at any moment. I had this 'bearing down' feeling and shooting pains up my vagina. I was really scared now. All this money had been spent, my business was in limbo and I had no money coming in. I was unable to work or care for my children. I was in worse pain and spent most of my days in the house, bed bound. I didn't know what would become of me.

As the symptoms progressed I emailed the consultant again and again. The consultant now informed me that he thought I had now developed another condition called adenomyosis; and started talking straight away about a hysterectomy. I was horrified he should immediately talk about a hysterectomy and not explore other options. I insisted on getting confirmation of this new condition, but he said it could only be done by an MRI scan. I decided that I would get my own MRI scan done after being told it would be another 12 weeks waiting time on NHS. Adenomyosis can often be classified with or misinterpreted as endometriosis, and can cause severe pelvic pain and menstrual irregularities. Adenomyosis occurs when nodules, or knots of endometrial tissue develop and grow into and within the smooth deep muscle layers of the uterus. Sadly the MRI confirmed that endometriosis was still in my pelvis and adenomyosis was evident so now I also had the added complication of adenomyosis.

My Diary Extract
Friday 29th April 2011, 01.02 am

"I am sat here in the kitchen crying and sobbing. I feel so utterly depressed, lonely, alone and a total big fat failure. I feel so weak and 'wabbit'. My tummy is in so much pain. I feel so scared and depressed. Why am I still ill? It has been over four months now. I feel there is no end in sight. What is to become of me I wonder? Is this it? Will I be ill, in pain, shuffling around, doubled over with a hot water bottle attached to my belly, forever? House and bed bound, a total home bird and social

recluse. I am sick of making plans and having to cancel them. I am sick of making excuses to people, and having to try and explain the pain. The unpredictability of endometriosis is so hard and the people I do see keep saying that I look ok! It makes me want to scream. I do not want to sound like I am feeling sorry for myself but I struggle to put a brave face on and to pretend my endometriosis is not tearing me up inside. I am finding it's easier to pretend that I am okay. I can see people thinking "is she making this up?" How on earth could you make up this living nightmare!? No one could make this up. Do people genuinely think anyone would choose the existence that I have right now? That is what it feels like, 'an existence'. It is a big struggle to get through each hour let alone each day. I keep hoping and praying for a way out; for someone to help me. Surely there must be another way, other than the touted 'cure' referred to as a hysterectomy. A hysterectomy is no cure, but a way of getting you out of the gynaecologist's ear... I feel lost in a dark, overgrown maze, suffocating in the cycle of the medical machine..."

The suggestion by the consultant to have a hysterectomy felt an extreme one. What was obvious to me however, was that once my uterus and ovaries were removed through a hysterectomy I would no longer be referred back to the gynaecological department as all 'gynaecological parts' would be removed. It felt like I was being passed along the well worn conveyor belt of the medical machine to be processed like a product and not a person. More importantly, a hysterectomy is not a cure for endometriosis and surely the consultant knew that?

It was time to re-evaluate other options that might be available to me.

Chapter 9

Surgery Side Effects

* * *

Hope springs eternal - Alexander Pope

I t was back to the drawing board for me. I took the

time to re-examine what had gone wrong and where I was currently. I looked again at the medical hormonal options being offered to me and what else the modern medical machine could offer me by way of surgical treatments, and it appeared to be a long list of invasive damaging side effects.

What I had come to realise was that surgery was not the 'quick fix' I had hoped for. In fact, it should have been the very last option, and only after I had done thorough research on the procedure to understand the risks and side effects and made sure I had a longer conversation with the surgeon. For instance, I learned that prior to any surgical procedure, your abdomen is covered with a anaesthetic substance which is used to try and sterilise the incision area. This substance can be toxic to our mitochondria (which are the little energy battery packs inside our cells). When our mitochondria have toxic substances inhibiting their function our bodies are less able to operate effectively and chronic fatigue may develop. Then during the operation the abdomen is inflated with carbon dioxide so the surgeon can get more accessibility for the instruments. These two substances alone can add additional toxic stress to an already ill body.

I learned that endometriosis can cause severe inflammation in the pelvic cavity which results in the formation of scar tissue referred to as adhesions. These adhesions are best compared to the thin white skin that can be seen on top of chicken breasts. When they form they can restrict organs in the pelvic area from moving and cause them to stick together and is referred to as a 'frozen pelvis'. And operations also cause more adhesions…

Endometriosis can grow into the layers of the tissue and interfere with the nerve endings. You may experience what appears to be unrelated pain but it can radiate up through into the back, legs and vulva. Tissues and cysts may fill with liquid which spill out over the organs and cause irritation, chronic and acute pain. And operations also irritate further nerve endings and organs…

When our body has an injury of any kind prostaglandins are released into the area to attack the offending 'enemy', by activating an inflammatory response. This process perpetuates the prolonged and continued agonising pain of women with endometriosis. The inflammatory issues still remain an issue after any operation but are aggravated by it.

Lets look at the range of invasive operations that are currently offered to women with endometriosis:

Diagnostic Laparoscopy
A diagnostic laparoscopy is used to confirm a suspected diagnosis of endometriosis and to evaluate the severity of the condition. During laparoscopy operation, the surgeon determines the number, size, and location of endometrial implants and adhesions: if they can be seen. In theory the surgeon is expected to drain any cysts, cut, burn or separate any adhesions but this does not always happen. Some

surgeons merely confirm 'diagnosis' of endometriosis implants and then finish the operation without the removal of endometrial implants.

The 'keyhole' surgical procedure involves a small incision in the abdomen and inserting a small thin fibre optic tube with a valve called a 'Trocar'. The laparoscope is equipped with a small telescopic lens, which enables the doctor view the uterus, ovaries, tubes, and peritoneum (lining of the pelvis) on a video monitor.

Although a laparoscopy is regarded as conservative surgery the side effects and risks are many and undertaking any operation should be taken seriously. The lasers that are expected to burn or cut adhesions can sometimes hit the bladder, bowel, uterus, ovaries, fallopian tubes and abdominal wall causing severe long term side effects.

Another big issue is the reoccurrence of adhesions and cysts soon after the surgery. As the body has been cut open and the internal organs moved about, cut and burnt, then the inflammatory and repair process in the body begin again. This means that adhesions that have just been cut may regrow during the bodies natural need to want to repair. The vicious cycle of operation, adhesions, operation, adhesions and operation continues. Put simply: endometriosis causes adhesions and operations cause adhesions.

I read about a woman who had 26 operations for her endometriosis, and not only did it not help her but made her worse. An operation is very damaging to a body that is already under stress and inflammation.

Laparotomy
A laparotomy is an operation where the surgeon makes a large incision into the abdomen. In some cases a laparoscopy can turn into a laparotomy if complications occur and a large access site is needed for the surgeon.

Laparoscopy Ablation and Excision

Ablation and excision laparoscopic operation is when the surgeon spends longer removing, scraping and cutting out what endometrial deposits, lesions, cysts or adhesions that can be seen. However, the operation does not prevent or limit the recurrence of lesions and symptoms. The operation is a traumatic experience for the body, and the reoccurrence of adhesions may occur within weeks. In addition there may be long-term bladder or bowel injury, or ovarian dysfunction.

Pre-Sacral-Neurectomy (PSN)

Pre-sacral-neurectomy is a procedure where the surgeon cuts the nerves that transmit the pain from your uterus to your brain. The surgeon has to cut through a numerous blood vessels. Evidence suggests that PSN carries high risk, is incomplete and is subject to controversy.

Laparoscopic Uterine Nerve Ablation (LUNA)

Laparoscopic uterine nerve ablation is when the surgeon cuts the sympathetic and para-sympathetic uterosacral nerves that transmit pain from uterus to the brain. Evidence suggests that LUNA carries high risk, is incomplete and like PSN, is subject to controversy.

Da Vinci Operation (Robot)

The Da Vinci robotic surgery is conducted by a robotic device. The very fact that a machine rather than a human being is carrying out the surgery means that there are major risks. The side effects can be devastating and there may be life-altering injuries from surgery complications, including burns, tears and other problems.

I felt I had reached a dead end, a no through road. What was I to do? I was still in excruciating pain. I was unable to leave the house, play with my children, go to work and my clients were moving on to new businesses. Many, if not all of the medical treatment options being suggested to me felt barbaric and had awful side effects. I had spent thousands of pounds trying the laparoscopy ablation and excision surgery route but it had failed. The surgeon had assured me that all of the adhesions, cysts and endometrial deposits would be removed and I would be back on my feet in now time. But I had got worse within weeks of the operation not better. What on earth was going on in my body?.

I found myself wrestling endlessly with my old beliefs that the medical profession was my only option and they had to 'fix' me. However I realised that to the 'medical machine' I was just a number and someone to process. The options I was being given didn't really feel like options at all, merely a life sentence to dependency on painkillers, hormonal drugs and surgery. That did not feel like a life for me.

Chapter 10 -

The Hysterectomy Hoax

* * *

God grant me the serenity to accept the things I cannot change, the courage to change the things I can, and the wisdom to know the difference
- Serenity Prayer

About 20 million woman in USA have had a

hysterectomy operation performed and by the age of 60 years old roughly a third of all women will have had one. Hysterectomy is the second most frequently performed surgical procedure with some 433,621 operations carried out per year in USA and roughly 55,000 in the UK. Clearly, as you can see, hysterectomy operations are BIG business in the Western world.

After a woman with endometriosis reaches a certain age or has had children, the most common suggestion by doctors is to have a hysterectomy. Yet very few women question the validity and necessity of this procedure. Your uterus is more than just a 'baby bag', as some doctors like to refer to it as. A hysterectomy operation is the removal of a woman's sex organs (the equivalent is removing a man's testicles and penis): female castration, and causes lifelong damage to the body.

In his book, 'The Hysterectomy Hoax', Dr Stephen West says that only 2% of hysterectomies are warranted; generally in the case of cancer. The uterus is an important organ that provides many hormones to prevent heart disease and osteoporosis; thinning of bones. A hysterectomy is **NOT** a cure for endometriosis, as any endometrial lesions or deposits that were in the abdominal cavity may still be there after the uterus has been removed.

Nora W. Coffey, who set up the Hysterectomy Education Resources and Services (HERS) Foundation and is the author of book called 'The H Word', offers advice and free information to women considering a hysterectomy. Nora has gathered evidence for over 10 years about the side effect to having a hysterectomy and she claims there are at least 170 different symptoms. I was very fortunate to speak with Nora personally and she informed me about all the risks. It was pretty hard to ignore them and go blindly on.

It became clear to me that despite the mounting pressure from my partner and the doctors to have a hysterectomy, it was not an option for me. Although, I almost did relent one day. The pain had become increasingly unbearable. I was sobbing and distraught, desperate for a way out. I could not take the pain any more. In an impulsive moment I tried to call the hospital to arrange the hysterectomy. I didn't want one but no other options were being presented to me. The telephone number rang out and out and out. It was normally a telephone that was answered immediately by an efficient team of secretaries. Fortunately for me that day it wasn't answered either time I called. An hour later I received a telephone call from Dian Shepperson Mills, the nutritionalist and author of the book 'Endometriosis: A Guide to Healing Through Nutrition'. I had been trying to contact her for a few days and as soon as I explained my situation she reassured me to hold firm. Dian reiterated the permanent damage a hysterectomy operation causes and to take charge, reexamine a few areas of my life the operation was not going to cure. My mother was never the same after her operation and talked of her great regret in having a hysterectomy carried out. I shall be forever grateful to Dian for telephoning me that day and saving my uterus.

A hysterectomy may 'appear' a tempting solution but it is not. The many severe side effects are rarely explained to women. Equally, women who have had a hysterectomy invariably fail to realise that the onset of new symptoms and problems they experience afterwards are due to the removal of her important sex organs.

After learning about the uterus's important structure and positioning in the body, I realised why a hysterectomy would cause new symptoms:

Uterus - The Heart of the South
The uterus (womb) is situated in the heart of the pelvis and is often referred to as the 'heart of the south'. It is positioned in-between, and keeps separate, the bladder and intestines. The removal of the uterus displaces these organs. Imagine a carefully designed architectural structure and the central part being removed. The surrounding areas all shift and move. There are three sets ligaments that are cut which hold the uterus in place and connect it to the cervix, floor and walls of the pelvis. These ligaments contain nerve endings which are sensitive to movement and play a role in pelvic pain if contorted by adhesions.

The uterus is best associated as the organ where a baby grows and unfortunately many doctors only view the organ for this purpose; sometimes referring to it as a 'baby bag'. The lining of the uterus is called the endometrium and provides nourishment for a growing baby. At the bottom of the uterus is the cervix which is a passage that leads to the vagina allowing for expulsion of menstrual flow and intake of sperm. When endometriosis is on the cervix it can cause pain on contact and tenderness. During sex when the penis enters the vagina it often contacts the cervix which causes pain or discomfort during sex and then in some cases bleeding.

Some doctors fail to realise the significance and importance of female sex organ and often suggest the removal of through a hysterectomy as a 'cure'. Without our uterus we will not be able to experience a female uterine orgasm - it is the equivalent of a man having his penis and testicles removed. The vagina is damaged, urinary incontinence, bone thinning and heart disease, weight gain are common consequences when the uterus is removed. It is worth repeating that a hysterectomy is NOT a cure for endometriosis, however appealing the doctors may make it sound to us the idea of having the 'troublesome' organ removed. Any endometriosis lesions in the abdomen will still continue to grow, shed and bleed in response to estrogen in the body. A hysterectomy causes life long damage to the body. Nora Covey mentioned in her book how her body was unable to float in the swimming pool, and kept tilting to the side, after her uterus was removed. This was an organ worth holding on to for many reasons.

Ovaries
Two oval shaped ovaries about the size of a large grape are positioned either side of the uterus and attached to fallopian tubes which lead to the uterus. Ovaries are responsible for the production of estrogen and progesterone, which are the two main hormones that are primarily involved in the woman's maturation of reproductive system and cyclic changes in the endometrium. The surgical removal of ovaries (oophorectomy or ovariectomy) along with the uterus, results in the women being thrown into immediate menopause which can be very severe and distressing consisting of hot flushes, brittle bones and HRT. The rate of complications and side effects are high, with the risk of death being about 1 in 1,000 women.

The Bladder

The bladder is a very sensitive organ that is positioned above the uterus. The urethra is a small tube that connects from the kidneys to the bladder. Sometimes, due to adhesions and endometriosis deposits, the tube can become bent or tangled, which in turn causes referred pain in the kidneys situated to the lower back region. Pressure and urgency to pee can be triggered too when endometriosis lesions are attached to the bladder. Many women experience increase in discomfort in their bladder and increased infections after a hysterectomy. This may be because the surgeon has touched or aggravated the bladder or bowel during the operation, and/or because the bladder now sits on top of the bowel where the uterus separated them before. Some women loose all bladder sensation for days or longer after surgery and require a catheter to be fitted. This can be particularly distressing for women whose bladder sensation never returns. The cutting of nerve endings and ligaments also cause more trauma and sensitivity to the bladder and bowel.

The Bowel

The bowel, (also be referred to as the intestines), is another organ that endometriosis tissue can implant itself on to. The bowel is a long muscular tube that is part of your digestive tract. The bowel extends from the low end of your stomach, down the small intestine into the large intestine, towards your back passage or anus. A high percentage of women with endometriosis suffer from bowel symptoms. They can include, and not be exclusive, to pain during bowel movements, changes in stool colour, blood in stools, constipation or diarrhoea. Adhesions can wrap around the bowel and if the surgeon makes contact with the bowel or 'nicks' it during surgery, the bowel can become affected and sensitivity may be increased.

Many side effects of hysterectomies are irreversible and cause life long damage. Nora Covey and Dian Shepperson Mills reminded me regularly of the consequences, as I wrestled with how to move forward. I was told how a hysterectomy may cause bladder incontinence (the uterus that had sat in-between separating the bladder and bowel has now gone) and a loss of uterine orgasm (you cannot have an orgasm if there is no uterus). Also how during the operation the vagina is shortened when the cervix and uterus are removed, and the top of the vagina is sewn up; theoretically it is turned into a 'pocket' which may prolapse (turns inside out). Once the uterus and ovaries are removed the body is then thrown into an immediate menopause. Although there would be no menstrual bleeding, any endometriosis left in my body would still grow. Ovaries even if left in during a hysterectomy (oophorectomy) would have reduced blood supply due to the cutting of blood vessels and nerves, and within 2 years, on average, another operation would be needed to remove them.

I realised that although I was impatient to get well, having a hysterectomy was like jumping from a chip pan into a fire. My mother had a hysterectomy and she was never the same afterwards. I saw there was no quick fix medical option; I would merely be swapping one set of problems for another. Once my important female organs were removed it was permanent. It would not be an option to get a transplant and get them replaced. When they were gone, they were gone. A hysterectomy was not an option as I could potentially double, if not triple, side effects and symptoms.

There had to be another way…

Chapter 11 -

Bad Affects of Estrogen Dominance

∗ ∗ ∗

Our deepest fear is not that we are inadequate. Our deepest fear is we are powerful beyond measure - Marianne Williamson

Sandra works full-time while raising three young children and she has been suffering from insomnia and night sweats, even though she is only in her early thirties and far away from entering into menopause; Kathlyn, a busy stockbroker, has such heavy periods that she is often locked in her house for seven days every month using the excuse of 'working from home'; and Patricia, newly married with an exciting job, is losing her hair, gaining weight around the middle, and always feeling exhausted. All three women are suffering from a common condition called Estrogen Dominance.

Nowadays, we are seeing girls reaching puberty as early as age eight. You go and ask any woman and chances are she is bound to say she has experienced Premenstrual Syndrome (PMS) at sometime in their life, and maybe even endometriosis, fibroids, or ovarian cysts. The common culprit in these conditions? Too much estrogen.

Every woman's body contains two main sex hormones, estrogen and progesterone. Estrogen is the female sex hormone and its counterpart in males is testosterone. Both hormones are present in both sexes. Estrogen includes three estrus-producing compounds: estrone, estradiol, and estriol. Estrogen is produced in a woman's body in small amounts by the ovaries, the adrenal cortex, the testes, and the fetoplacental unit.

What is the role that estrogen plays in our bodies then? In women, estrogen plays an important role in the growth and development of female secondary sexual characteristics such as breasts, armpit and pubic hair, endometrium, regulation of the reproductive system and the menstrual cycle. Every menstrual cycle, estrogen produces an environment suitable for fertilisation, implantation, and nutrition of the embryo.

In males, estrogen also plays an important role for normal male reproduction and assists in maturation of the sperm cells. Pubertal development in boys, such as growing long bones, are attributed to the actions of androgens, however, it is now recognised as being mediated in part by estrogen.

What does estrogen do in women? Estrogen is a very important component and it contributes to a woman's menstrual cycle and ability to bear children. I will show below how estrogen affects the vital organs of the female reproductive system:

- **Ovaries** – estrogen mainly helps stimulate the growth of the egg follicle.
- **Vagina** – estrogen stimulates the growth of the vagina to its adult size. Estrogen also thickens the vaginal wall and increases the vaginal acidity to reduce the risk of bacterial infections.
- **Fallopian tubes** – estrogen keeps maintenance of the endometrium, the mucus membrane that lines the insides of the uterus. Estrogen is responsible for

increasing the endometrium's size and weight, the number of cells, types of cells, flow of blood, protein content, and enzyme activity. Estrogen is also responsible for stimulating the muscles in the uterus to develop and contract. These contractions are vital as these help the uterine wall to cast off dead tissue during menstruation and during delivery of a child and the placenta.

- **Cervix** – estrogen regulates the flow and thickness in the uterine mucus secretions to enhance the transport of the sperm cells.
- **Mammary glands** – estrogen unifies with other hormones in the female breasts. It is responsible for the growth of the female breasts during adolescence and the pigmentation of the nipples.

Let us delve further into the process by which estrogen plays its role during a menstrual cycle. Estrogen controls the menstrual cycle and the amount of it in a woman's body which naturally rises and falls throughout the month.

Day 1 of the cycle
Estrogen and progesterone levels at this point in the cycle are at their lowest.

Day 5 of the cycle
An egg is selected. Inside the ovary, the egg is contained within a follicle and the anatomic structure where the egg develops. The follicle will begin to release increasing amounts of estrogen.

Days 6 to 13 of the cycle
Preparing for ovulation. From this point and toward the end of this stage, estrogen levels will rise slowly and then, will rise more rapidly.

Day 14 of the cycle

The follicle that contains the egg will break open and the ovary will release the egg into the fallopian tube. It will stay there and wait for sperm to fertilise it. The follicle will remain in the fallopian tube.

Days 15 to 28 of the cycle

After ovulation. At this stage, the levels of progesterone will start to increase. If the egg waiting in the fallopian tube is not fertilised, both estrogen and progesterone levels will drop after two weeks and the lining of the insides of the uterus gets ready to be shed. At this point, menstruation begins, and the cycle will start all over again.

Our menstrual cycle is a very dynamic process that repeats itself every 28 days on average and you can clearly see that estrogen plays a role that is important to the whole process. We women are all too familiar with mood changes and disturbances during our periods, and estrogen is thought to be involved.

If estrogen is good for our body, why is it bad to have too much of it? In women, the normal levels of progesterone and estrogen should exist in a ratio of 30 to 1. When that ratio is skewed, a woman's body becomes deficient in progesterone or excessive in estrogen; either way the woman goes to a state of 'estrogen dominance'. Apart from reproduction, estrogen influences many of the other physiological processes in a woman's body, such as cardiovascular health, bone integrity, cognition, and behaviour. With this extensive role, it is not surprising that estrogen is also implicated in the development or progression of numerous diseases. This is the reason why we women should always keep estrogen levels in check.

Among the diseases that excess estrogen is closely responsible for are breast cancer, ovarian cancer, colorectal cancer, heart disease, neurodegenerative diseases, Alzheimer's disease,

Parkinson's disease, gallstones, osteoporosis, Systemic Lupus Erythematosus (SLE), and our main concern, endometriosis, which, if left unchecked, can potentially lead to endometrial cancer.

How do we know if we are in a state of estrogen dominance? Here is a list of common symptoms to watch out for in estrogen dominance and endometriosis:

- Unusually painful periods, heavy bleeding, or clots
- Pelvic pain
- Sore, swollen, tender breasts and nipples
- Irregular periods or unusually long periods
- Premenstrual syndrome (PMS) or premenstrual tension (PMT)
- Ovarian cysts
- Abnormal pap smear
- Migraines & head fog
- Fat gain around hips, stomach, and thighs
- Water retention
- Puffiness
- Bloating
- Hair thinning and hair loss
- Chronic fatigue
- Insomnia
- Hot flashes, burning up and night sweats
- Restless legs at night
- Excessively weepy close to your cycle
- Low thyroid function
- Lower back pain
- Painful bowel movements
- Bladder pressure and frequency

If you are experiencing 2 or more of the above symptoms then you could have a pretty serious hormonal imbalance happening.

Extreme cases of estrogen dominance can also be seen when there are symptoms like:

o   Fibroids
o   Uterine cancer
o   Ovarian cancer
o   Breast cancer

I admit to knowing very little about how my body functioned and even less about my hormonal cycle at this time. I had heard about progesterone and estrogen but was unaware of how an imbalance could have such an impact on our bodies. Estrogen dominance was a phrase that I could finally identify with. I now understood why, despite having removed wheat and sugar from my diet, I was still in pain.

I had a severe hormonal imbalance that needed to be looked at in greater detail.

Chapter 12 -

Our Toxic World

* * *

A journey of a thousand miles begins with a single step - Confucius

My research led me to understand the term 'estrogen dominance' better and also, taught me that endometriosis and adenomyosis were estrogen dominant conditions. If we already have enough estrogen produced in our body, why do we still get more, and why does it cause estrogen dominance? Most of you women out there may not be aware of this reality and I think this is the right time to let you know. This was a wakeup call and also, a turning point in my healing.

Every day of our lives, environmental estrogens bombard us and we are blind to it. They are called 'xenoestrogens' or estrogen mimickers. These fabricated estrogen chemicals are imposters acting exactly like the estrogen in our bodies. These estrogen mimickers are found in almost everything, from plastics, chemicals in cosmetics, pesticides, washing powders, dry cleaning chemicals, the pollution in our environment, even food and dairy products, and so much more. If we constantly expose ourselves to all of these, we will be susceptible to additional estrogen absorption, and too much estrogen will upset the body's delicate balance of hormones.

Other sources of estrogen that we may unknowingly take are beef and meats that were grown and fed with antibiotics and growth hormones. Soy or soya, which, by nature, already contains plant-based estrogens, referred to as 'phytoestrogens'.

Medications, such as birth control pills or oral contraceptives and intrauterine devices like coils, also contribute to estrogen dominance. Birth control pills prevent the ovulation of the egg cell, and as I described above, estrogen plays a lead role in ovulation. Therefore, if ovulation is prevented, it leaves estrogen with nothing else to do but increase in levels, and this is clearly not good. If you do not ovulate you do not produce progesterone as you would do if you released an egg every month. Overtime, no ovulation may create a serious progesterone deficiency. Although there are many medical, social, and emotional reasons why women take birth control pills, it might be a good time to reconsider using other forms of contraceptive like condoms or femidoms, or fertility awareness-based methods (FAMs) which are ways to track ovulation in order to prevent pregnancy.

Processed foods are also full of excess estrogens that our body does not need. Always go organic and fresh for your choices of food as much as possible. Also, keep tabs on your body weight. Our own body will naturally compensate and add estrogen for every pound of weight we gain. Therefore, it is definitely not very advisable to go beyond your ideal weight.

Too much alcohol and too much coffee can also contribute to estrogen dominance in our bodies. Alcohol, for one, can weaken our liver. As we all know, our liver is our body's filter and is the key for detoxification, especially with excess hormones. When we do not eat a well-balanced diet and take on too much of one thing (such as fats, sugars, or alcohol) and not enough vegetables and good protein, this makes our liver sluggish and congested, and unable to function fast enough to eliminate these toxins. Once that happens, the hormones will be left unchecked and this will create a hormonal imbalance.

Xenoestrogens

Some synthetic chemicals mimic and disrupt the hormonal balance in women. They do this by blocking or binding receptors and because they are not biodegradable they get stored in our fat cells.

Studies have shown that women produce 50% less progesterone at age 20-35 compared to our ancestors. This may be because of chemical and toxin exposures. The rise in estrogen mimickers may also be why there are many young girls entering puberty prematurely. Men's sperm count has also decreased by 50% in some industrial parts of the world. Scientists have also found some fish downstream from sewage treatment plants to have changed sex from male to female due to the estrogen in the water.

Tap drinking water has been found to contain a primary estrogen compound that is in birth control pills called ethynylestadiol (EE) so consider getting a house water filter or drink mineral water.

One chemical that is particularly harmful is called Glyphosate which is used as a herbicide. Glyphosate has been shown by France's University of Caen to potential cause fertility problems, miscarriages and abnormal foetal development.

Genetically Modified Food

Genetically modified foods (GMO) first came on the market in 1994 with soybean, corn, canola, cottonseed oil, sugar and aspartame being some of the main products. Although GMO's were designed to be resistant to bugs, disease and drought and have a longer shelf life. However, they have been shown to cause harm to humans and animals. It has been estimated that at least 70% of processed foods contain at least one genetically modified ingredient and are causing estrogen dysregulation.

I had not realised just how toxic our environment was. I felt irritated that I had been so trusting of global brand name products and had never even thought to question what was put in my body, on my body or around my body. If many of these personal care and household products were so toxic then why were we not fully informed that putting them in our bodies could make us so ill?

I also wanted to know what I could do to remove these toxins from my life.

Chapter 13 -

Fighting Against the Toxins

* * *

Courage is not the absence of fear, but rather the judgment that something else is more important than fear - Ambrose Redmoon

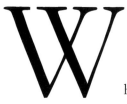hat are the ways to fight against the environmental toxins, rebalance your hormones, and prevent estrogen dominance?

Firstly, the liver, thyroid, and the adrenal glands must operate at peak performance to ensure good hormonal balance and harmony. The best way to achieve this is to employ a good diet program and elimination of toxins that are poisoning your body. The liver is the largest internal organ inside the body, although it is often considered the second largest to the skin. The liver is an important organ and has many functions, but the main one is to expel toxins that are ingested into the body. The long term use of pain killers are toxic to the liver and may have an adverse effect on its ability to rid the body of excess estrogens.

Hormone-Free Food
Eat only organic, grass fed, hormone free meat and poultry as much as possible. Try to get hold of meat from wild and free-range livestock to obtain the best lean protein. Avoid all non-organic meats, dairy, refined sugar, vegetable oils, refined

flours, and carbohydrates which are full of E numbers, additives and preservatives.

No Wheat

One type of food, as I have pointed out in the previous chapters, is the removal of wheat from your diet. A sign that your body has a wheat intolerance can be if you find your stomach gets bloated and distended after eating it. Wheat is genetically modified and is very hard on the digestive track. Try an exclusion diet for three months and then reintroduce it to see the effects. Eat plenty of fibre rich vegetables and focus specially on the cruciferous ones like kale, broccoli, cauliflower, cabbage, hok choy, and brussels sprouts to name a few. Broccoli comes highly recommended because it contains indole-3 carbinole (I3C), which helps in detoxifying estrogen out of the body.

No Coffee

Stop drinking coffee which has been proven to increase estrogen in the body by a staggering 73%! Try a delicious alternative called Roobius or Red Bush tea instead. It is naturally caffeine free and very tasty.

No Plastics or Microwavables

Avoid using the microwave or heating food in plastic materials.and consider replacing any plastic kettles with stainless steel ones. A study showed that plastic cling film or wrap, that is heated in a microwave has 500,000 times the minimum amount of xenoestrogens needed to stimulate and grow breast cancer cells in a test tube. Quite shocking figures!

Personal Products & Cosmetics

Clean up your environment. Get rid of all the unnecessary cosmetics especially those with ingredients that you **cannot** pronounce; that is a sign it is not natural. Minimise, if not stop, applying lotions on your skin even if only temporarily ,whilst you are unwell and in chronic pain. These contain xenoestrogens, parabens, and sodium laurel sulphates

(SLS) which are toxic chemicals which your skin will absorb directly into the bloodstream. Cheap brands tend to have more chemicals in them so are best avoided. One natural, and inexpensive approach I have tried and still use today, is coconut oil, rice bran oil, and shea butter. They give the same effect of smoothing your skin but best of all, they are 100% natural. A lot of the creams have these natural products as bases and then load the chemicals on top. Use organic non perfumed shampoos or soap bars, and avoid nail varnish and nail polish removers as they are highly toxic. Use natural paraben-free sunscreen lotions. I like using olive oil, which gives my skin good protection and a lovely colour.

Tampons
Only use organic tampons. Many tampons and sanitary pads have bleach in them which can cause allergic toxic reactions. Toxic Shock Syndrome (TSS) is a rare but serious and sometimes fatal disease, where the body's response to the poisons (the bacteria called Staphylococcus Aureus or Staph) is to go into shock. This can be seen to affects those who use super-absorbent tampons. Never leave tampons in for more than three hours and **NEVER** overnight. Why not try a 'Mooncup' which is a reusable menstrual cup about 2" long. It is greener, safer and cheaper than the chemically laden tampons or sanitary towels. Worn internally, the Mooncup catches the menstrual fluid, becomes leak-free, and can be worn for hours.

Household Products
For your cleaning around the house, use green cleaning products, or better yet, make your own. There are hundreds of 'do-it-yourself' cleaning product recipes, and you can find them on the internet. Most of them use simple ingredients like bicarbonate soda and vinegar that can be found already in your home. It is important to change your washing powder, as clothes washed in chemical laden products continue to release these chemicals when worn. Swap out with coconut based products There are many suppliers online which offer a

great selection and many deliver worldwide. Do not use fabric softeners or tumble dryer sheets ,as petrochemicals are used in them and they sit right on top, being directly absorbed into your skin.

Invest in a Good Water Filter

Invest in a good quality water filter for the house or a water filter jug. The consumption of birth control pills and other synthetic hormones contribute to estrogen contaminating the streams, rivers and waterway systems. Drink water from glass bottles only, and if a plastic water container has been heated up, do **NOT** drink the water and throw it away immediately.

Detox

Detoxify your liver at least twice a year. I was able to achieve this by eating nothing but fresh free range food for a month, practising regular vegetable juicing, and using Chlorella cracked cell powder. I can clearly observe the positive effects because of the resulting light and energetic feeling I get afterwards. However, a word of caution: women with endometriosis need to get out of pain first and have enough energy before they can consider about doing a detox. Detoxing is exhausting on the body the first few times. and your body needs to be strong and have energy for the process. Remember, we are going to be healing gently, so go slowly before thinking about doing this.

Regular Bowel Movements

Try as much as possible to practice regular bowel movements. After your liver detoxifies, it sends all the excess estrogen hormones to the stool to be excreted from your body once you poop. You are looking to discharge waste matter from the large intestine and out of the body at least once a day. If by some misfortune you are constipated, the stool becomes immobile, and the estrogens and other toxins can be reabsorbed through the intestines and back into your system. You definitely do not want that. Therefore, drink eight glasses of fresh mineral water a day and eat vegetables full of fibre to keep your bowel movements regular to facilitate good detoxification.

Get a Good Night's Sleep

Getting a good night's sleep is easier said than done for women with endometriosis. In fact more often than not, that was when the pain would escalate. If you find yourself having difficulty getting to sleep, try taking a natural sleeping aid containing melatonin, hops, chamomile, valerian and passionflower. This worked wonders for me and really helped me a lot. If you are finding it hard to sleep due to the pain, lie with your feet elevated, eyes closed, focusing on your breathing, which will help to get your body into a restful and healing state. I used to get quite stressed when I was not able to sleep, but I learnt that lying down and listening to 'bilateral' relaxing music helped me to focus on my breath, enabling my body to get into a healing state. Your overworked adrenal glands need the sleep or deep rest. When your body releases adrenaline, you will feel exhaustion quickly once the effects of the hormone fade out. You can reverse this by getting proper sleep or deep restful periods of at least eight hours a day.

Happy Thyroid

Keep your thyroid glands healthy. Both the adrenal glands and thyroid glands are directly linked, so once the adrenals get exhausted, the thyroid also goes low. Pay a visit to your doctor to get them checked if you suspect that your thyroid does not function well enough. Swap your regular toothpaste for a fluoride-free one as studies have shown that fluoride interferes with the thyroid function. The Food and Drug Administration (FDA) has acknowledged potential risks and requires a poison warning on every tube of toothpaste now sold in the USA!

When I first learned about all of the toxic ingredients in my food, personal and household products I felt quite overwhelmed and unsure where to start. It was also no wonder I had been so increasingly ill if all of these toxins were poisoning my body, and perpetuating a severe hormonal imbalance and estrogen dominance.

I appreciate that at first read of the above it might feel like a BIG adjustment to your life: but it is worth it. These products are making you ill and keeping you ill. Endometriosis is 'fed' and inflamed every time you apply a product that is a xenoestrogen. Start by making small adjustments, as you can afford them, but it is important to increase your awareness of what goes in your body, on your body and is around your body.

Chapter 14 -

The Power of Bio-Identical Progesterone Cream

* * *

Minds are like parachutes; they only function when they are open
- Thomas Dewar

I have described in the earlier chapters how the

two main sex hormones, progesterone and estrogen, must maintain an ideal ratio of 30 to 1 or a woman's body goes into a state of estrogen dominance. Back in the 1970s, there existed a common fundamental misunderstanding about the physiological role of estrogen and progesterone over the course of a woman's reproductive life cycle. This resulted in a treatment strategy mostly for menopausal women, which was not based upon scientific evidence. Synthetic estrogen was so idealised back then and progesterone neglected. This led to significant suffering for premenopausal, perimenopausal and postmenopausal women. Studies have shown that for many women who suffered from these uncomfortable and often disabling symptoms, the mistake of supplementing with synthetic estrogen only aggravated their conditions.

I came to the realisation, once I had removed all xenoestrogens, that a decrease in progesterone and a significant increase in estrogen (estrogen dominance), is the real culprit behind these disorders in the female reproductive system. The medical establishments identified this and discovered a way to boost the progesterone deficiency from the synthetically pharmaceutically produced progesterone called 'Progestin' and 'Progestrone' (note how similar the names are to progesterone, which add to the confusion for women). Even though they start off using natural progesterone the pharmaceutical companies chemically alter it, but not identically to what we produce naturally in our bodies. This means they can patent the tablets and then sell them to medical establishments and hospitals. It is the chemical alteration which causes the number of unpleasant side effects.

However, many women have learned to use a natural bio-identical progesterone cream alternative to treat endometriosis. Natural bio-identical cream used to be routinely prescribed by doctors in USA and UK in the 1960's, before the pharmaceutical giants exercised their influence. This treatment regime is among the top choices that help reduce symptoms and aid in the treatment of endometriosis. When applied in a high enough dose, this treatment can induce a safe pseudo-pregnancy-like condition that actually helps stop the further development of endometriosis. The main objective of the bio-identical progesterone is to counteract the estrogen dominance. Using bio-identical progesterone cream also reduces further proliferation of endometriosis implants and also allow any other implants that are present to shrink. There are no known side effects from taking bio-identical progesterone cream, except for sleepiness when taken in great excess.

Hormone Testing
I would suggest getting a saliva hormone test done which is more reliable than a blood test. You may ask your doctor or order the testing kits, which are inexpensive, and can be purchased online. Test for estradiol and progesterone to determine a baseline to give yourself a comparison for the future. There are five ways that estrogen dominance can show up; high estrogen to low progesterone (which is the classic

definition of the imbalance), high estrogen to normal progesterone, normal estrogen to low progesterone, low estrogen to low progesterone and normal levels of estrogen and normal levels of progesterone. Whatever the results, if you are experiencing all of the classic estrogen dominant and endometriosis symptoms, it is because your body is being bombarded by many estrogen mimicking chemicals in our environment.

How to Use Natural Bio-identical Progesterone Cream

The proper procedure to use bio-identical progesterone cream is to apply it from day six of the cycle up until day 26, using one ounce of the cream per week, for three weeks, and then stop just before your expected period. After four to six months of use, you should be noticing that your menstrual pains have gradually subsided, because the monthly bleeding from the endometriosis implants is less and the healing of the inflammatory sites begin to occur.

You may wonder where do these bio-identical hormones come from? In the human body, the ovaries, the testicles, and the adrenal glands manufacture a series of hormones known as steroids that are all derived from cholesterol. In the early 1960s, science was able to synthesise all of these molecules starting either from cholesterol or from plant steroids found in nature. Bio-identical hormones are derived from a plant oil called diosgenin, which has a very similar chemical structure to cholesterol. Diosgenin is extracted primarily from wild yams and some bean species, but is also found in thousands of other plants worldwide. However, the human body cannot convert this compound into steroid hormones. Diosgenin needs to be chemically altered in a laboratory to exactly match the human steroid hormones. The manufactured molecules now exactly match the chemical structure and the effects of hormones that occur naturally in the human body, hence they are called bio-identical.

The Safe Hormone

Bio-identical progesterone contains the identical chemical structure and composition to the actual progesterone hormone produced in a woman's body. Bio-identical progesterone should not be confused with synthetic progesterone-like chemicals called progestins as mentioned earlier, because these are totally unnatural to a woman's body. These progestins bind to the body's progesterone receptors and function like progesterone but only temporarily. This happens because progestins are chemically different from bio-identical progesterones. They possess inherent side effects that may cause more harm than good to your already worsening endometriosis situation.

When you go to find a bio-identical progesterone cream, make sure you buy the ones with at least 500 mg of natural progesterone per ounce. So shop around, do enough research, and buy the best quality bio-identical progesterone cream you can afford for the treatment of your endometriosis condition. In the UK, some doctors can often prescribe a progesterone cream, like Emerita, if they are fund holding practises or if the Area Health Authority will pay.

Upon application, rub the cream on the parts of your body that have good circulation such as the breasts, neck, legs, chest, arms, thighs, soles of the feet, and the back. If you have a lot of body fat, the progesterone will be soaked up by that body fat first, before being absorbed into your blood stream. This means you will have to apply a higher dose to make it effective.

What should you do if you start to feel an increase in estrogen dominance symptoms after applying bio-identical progesterone cream? Experts would say that the introduction of progesterone may temporarily stimulate the body's estrogen receptor sites. As we all know, progesterone is the direct counterpart of estrogen, and it is normal for estrogen to react when progesterone is first introduced. If your bio-identical progesterone cream seems to have no affect on your condition, the most obvious answer to this is a poor quality product or dosage needs to be increased. If you have been using your bio-identical progesterone cream for more than 30 days as recommended and you do not see any improvement in your symptoms, then, this is unusual and you should consider changing your brand. Also, have another look around your personal and household products to see what xenoestrogens or phytoestrogens might still be lurking around and affecting your body.

I had made a conscious effort to remove all known toxins from my personal and household products and the application of natural bio-identical progesterone cream made a tremendous difference to my body and still does today. Combined with a few other factors, which I will be explaining in later chapters, natural bio-identical progesterone cream helped with the reduction of many of the endometriosis symptoms including; breast pain, stomach cramps, reduction in blood flow and premenstrual syndrome. And the best part of it all: it was all natural, compatible with my body and there were no side affects!

I was back in the driving seat of my body...

Chapter 15 -

The Endometriosis Power Protein Shake

* * *

The only thing you have to fear is fear itself
- Franklin D Roosevelt

I t is normal for women with endometriosis to look at

protein shakes and get the impression that these nutritious drinks are only for men or bodybuilders. In fact, a woman's body does not produce enough testosterone to build muscle in the same way as a man's body. Although, it is true that high-protein shakes help develop lean muscle mass, which can be a benefit for women. It is also true that these shakes actually encourage fat loss, increase satiety, deliver essential nutrients, improve energy, and metabolic activity.

Protein is known as the building blocks of our body alongside amino acids. Protein is vital in maintaining our body tissue, including development and repair of our hair, our skin, our eyes, and our muscles and organs, which are all made from protein. This is the main reason why children need more protein per pound of body weight than us adults. They are growing and developing new tissue.

Let us get a better understanding of the role of protein in our body. Protein is a very important substance found in every cell in the human body. In fact, other than water, protein is the most abundant substance in our body. This protein is manufactured by our body utilising the dietary protein we consume. Protein is used in many vital processes in our body and thus needs to be consistently replaced. We can accomplish this by regularly consuming foods that are rich in protein.

Protein is one of the major sources of energy for our body. If we consume more protein than we need for body tissue maintenance and other functions, our body will use it for energy.

Interestingly protein is very much involved in creating hormones. Proteins help control body functions that involve the interaction of several organs. For example, insulin, a small protein hormone, helps regulate blood sugar which interacts with organs such as the pancreas and the liver. Another example of a protein hormone, secretin, assists in the digestive process by stimulating the pancreas and the intestines to create the necessary digestive juices.

Protein is a major factor in transporting certain molecules inside our body. Haemoglobin, for example, is a protein that transports oxygen throughout our body. Apart from transportation, protein also acts as storage for certain molecules. Another example is ferritin, which combines with iron for storage in the liver.

Another magnificent role that protein plays in our body is the formation of antibodies. Antibodies help prevent infection, illness and disease. These proteins are the ones that identify and assist in destroying antigens, such as bacteria and viruses. These proteins often work in conjunction with the other immune system cells. First these antibodies will identify the intruders and then surround them in order to keep them contained, until they can be destroyed by the white blood cells.

Boost your body

The problem with a lot of women with endometriosis is that they are in such chronic pain that they lose their appetites and do not feel like eating. I often used go through the whole day without having breakfast or lunch, and wonder why at 3 pm I felt ill and tired! I would graze on sugar and chocolate to get energy hits (which releases dopamine; a feel-good feeling in the brain) to help me get through the rest of the day.

Now we know how important it is to maintain enough proteins in our body. If, for some reason, you cannot get enough protein from solid food, protein shakes are your best alternative to supplement your protein deficiency. There are so many different kinds of protein shakes sold in the market, but the essential ones that you should look out for are organic and non-genetically modified, or ideally make them yourself. Make sure to avoid whey or soy or sweeteners, and ideally consume organic rice or pea protein powder.

Replacing your meals with protein shakes, whilst you recover, can help you consume the calories and nutrients your body needs to repair and heal. It can also give you the energy your body needs to function in a day. You will eventually want to start eating solid food again once the pain reduces, but in the meantime, you may find it easier to 'drink' your food.

Aim to have at least one protein shake every day. Within one hour of waking make a protein shake consisting of one litre glass of water, juice or coconut milk, two tablespoons of rice or pea organic protein powder (i.e. non-GM), crush 2 good quality multi-vitamin and mineral tablets or use a rice based multi-vitamin and mineral powder, and top it up with nutritious green powder, like chlorella or spirulina that must be wheat free.

As you are recovering, I personally encourage you to combine protein shakes into your diet because of the numerous benefits these can give you. Always make sure that there are no wheat and added sugar in the ingredients. Whenever possible, it is still best to make your own protein shakes from fresh ingredients. This will keep you away from 'synthetic' ingredients included in off-the-shelf protein shakes sold in the supermarkets.

When you do start to eat solid proteins again please ensure they are good quality, hormone free, grass fed, and free range meat and poultry. Protein has had a lot of bad press over the years and alternatives like 'Quorn' and tofu have sprung up, but they are poor alternatives to animal protein, fish, pulses, beans, nuts, and seeds.

I had been totally ignorant about the vital role of protein for the healing of our bodies. I realised that the only food sources our cavemen and women ancestors would have lived off for thousands of years, would have been protein, nuts, seeds and fruit. Our Western society has expanded so rapidly over the past 80 years that governments have had to adjust to feeding the population easily and readily: hence the development of genetically modified foods and growth of wheat and soy products.

I suddenly saw food in a whole new light and it didn't seem so complicated after all and the best part was there were no nasty side affects. It was bye bye the bakers and hello nature...

Chapter 16 -

The Use of Multi-Vitamin and Mineral Supplements

* * *

You gain strength, courage and confidence by every experience in which you really stop to look fear in the face - Eleanor Roosevelt

There may be instances where you cannot get full access to all the best sources of nutrients through a well-balanced diet of protein power shakes or solid food. In this case, your other option is to introduce vitamins and mineral supplements to augment what is lacking from your diet.

We are what we eat, but why does what we eat these days lack the nutrition content we so badly need? Many of the foods we consume in the Western world have travelled great distances and are not grown locally. Those foods that do travel are picked early and are sprayed with pesticides to stop the ripening process. Some foods are genetically modified meaning they lack natural nutrients that we need to get from them.

Many women with endometriosis have nutritional deficiencies and require supplementation in the short to medium term. Iron deficiencies are common for those with a history of prolonged blood loss over many years. Ask your doctor to check your ferritin iron levels and even if they come back within range, but are on the low side, consider taking a non-constipating iron supplement every day for 3 months. This has shown to improve hair thickness and energy levels.

To replenish your body's nutrients, which help it heal more quickly, take a good quality (without talc) multi-vitamin and mineral tablet(s) or powder every day. Please get the best quality you can afford as the cheap versions are filled with nasty bulking agents. Other supplements worth considering are as follows:

Magnesium

Magnesium is a mineral that is present in relatively large amounts in our body. Estimates show that an average person's body contains 25 grams of magnesium; half of which are in the bones. Magnesium is vital in more than 300 chemical reactions that keep our body working. It is required for the proper growth and maintenance of our bones. It is also responsible for the proper function of our nerves, muscles, and many other parts of our body. In the stomach, for example, it helps neutralise stomach acid and moves stools conveniently through the intestine. A sign you may be deficient in magnesium is a constant craving for chocolate. Chocolate has high levels of magnesium in it; hence, that is why some people desire it. Restless, itchy, and unsettled sensations in the legs, especially in the night, can also be an indication of magnesium deficiency and estrogen dominance.

Zinc

Zinc is a metal and called an 'essential trace element' because only very small amounts of it are necessary for human health. It is essential for enzyme activity, helping cells to reproduce which eventually helps with healing processes. Therefore, zinc plays a vital role in our immune system. Moreover, Zinc is present in high concentrations in our eyes and is involved in maintaining good vision. Zinc is a catalyst for 100 enzymes in the body. Common signs that signal your body is low in zinc include slowed growth, loss of appetite, low insulin levels, irritability, generalised hair loss, slow wound healing, rough and dry skin, poor sense of taste and smell, diarrhoea, and nausea. Zinc Picolinate is best for absorption. A daily intake of Zinc is required as the body has no specialised way of storing it in the body.

Calcium

When our menstrual period draws near the calcium levels in our body decreases. This creates a calcium deficiency that can lead to muscle cramps, headaches, and pelvic pain. Calcium is a mineral that is a vital part of our bones and teeth. Our heart, nerves, and blood-clotting systems require calcium to work properly. Calcium helps to relieve premenstrual syndrome, leg cramps, high blood pressure, and reducing the risk of colon and rectal cancers. Our bones and teeth contain over 99% of the calcium present in our body. It is also found in the blood, muscles and other tissues. Calcium in our bones acts as a reserve and is released in the body when it is needed. This process occurs mostly in women during pregnancy, as the unborn infant is also supplied with calcium in the womb. As we age, the calcium concentration in our body declines because it is released through sweat, skin cells, and waste. Our bones are constantly breaking down and rebuilding, so we need to take extra calcium supplements to help to stay strong. Calcium D-Glucarate is best, as it has been shown to enhance the major detoxification in the body and decrease toxicity of xeno-estrogens in the bowel, as it promotes excretion.

Iron

Iron is a mineral and most of it is found in the haemoglobin of the red blood cells and in the myoglobin of muscle cells. Iron is responsible for transporting oxygen and carbon dioxide Iron does this by helping red blood cells deliver oxygen from the lungs to the cells all over our body. Once the oxygen is delivered, iron again helps the red blood cells carry carbon dioxide back to the lungs to be exhaled. Women with endometriosis who suffer from very heavy periods and excessive blood loss, can develop an iron deficiency causing them to become anaemic. This can mainly be characterised by a pale pallor, extreme fatigue and weakness.

Selenium

Selenium is a mineral and most of it in our body comes from our diet. The amount of selenium consumed depends on where in the world we live. Examples of good selenium sources are crabs, liver, fish, and poultry. The amount of selenium available varies widely, meaning that fish found in Europe will contain different levels of selenium from fish found in Asia, even though it can be the same species of fish. Selenium is used for diseases relating to the heart and blood vessels, including a stroke and the 'hardening of the arteries'. Selenium also seems to increase the action of antioxidants. Researchers have reported that selenium, when taken together with vitamin E, decreased the inflammation associated with the endometriosis condition.

B Vitamins

These vitamins are important for the breakdown of proteins, carbohydrates, and fats in our body. Research also showed that B vitamins helped in improving the emotional symptoms of women who have endometriosis and are responsible for energy metabolism, for a normal functioning nervous system and the reduction of tiredness and fatigue. One very important B vitamin is folic acid. All of the doctors in the world recommend that any woman of childbearing age must take folic acid supplement. The main reason is folic acid can protect against birth defects that may form before a woman knows she is pregnant. Another important B vitamin is vitamin B12 or better known as Cobalamin. Vitamin B12 plays a role in producing DNA and helps keep our nerve cells and red blood cells healthy. Vitamin B3, or non-flush Niacinamide, is another B vitamin that is good for your body. In order to be in good health it is vital to have large quantities of Niacinamide in our body. When used as a treatment, higher amounts of B3 can improve cholesterol levels and lower the risks of cardiovascular complications. B7, or Biotin, is particularly good for restoring hair loss and thickening hair. B vitamins are also water soluble so any excess that gets consumed will get flushed out of the body through urination and sweat glands.

Vitamin C

Vitamin C, or ascorbic acid, is the most well-known immune system booster and great for wound healing. Most experts still recommend getting vitamin C from a diet rich in fruits and vegetables for example freshly-squeezed orange juice. Our body also uses vitamin C to build and maintain collagen. Since Vitamin C is a water soluble vitamin and the body will extract its own requirements with any excess being flushed out in the urine or sweat glands.

Vitamin A

This is another well-known supplement for boosting our immune system. This vitamin is easily found in many fruits, vegetables, eggs, whole milk, butter, meat, and oily saltwater fish. Vitamin A helps women who experience heavy menstrual periods, premenstrual syndrome, vaginal infections, 'lumpy' breasts, and breast cancer. Pregnant and breast-feeding women who are diagnosed with HIV take vitamin A to decrease the risk of transmitting the HIV to the baby.

Vitamin E

The main benefits of vitamin E is its capability as an antioxidant. This means that it helps to slow down the processes that age and damage our cells. Vitamin E helps the distribution and oxygen carrying capacities of our haemoglobin. This is the reason why we see women who look 30 even when they are actually 50 years old. They have sufficient concentrations of vitamin E within their system. Vitamin E is also used to lessen the harmful effects of medical treatments such as dialysis and radiation. People who take medication for hair loss and lung damage can be seen to consume vitamin E to reduce unwanted side effects. Complications in late pregnancy, due to high blood pressure, premenstrual syndrome, very painful periods, menopausal syndrome, hot flashes and breast cysts, can be prevented by taking vitamin E.

Fish Oil

Fish oils offer many benefits and are important for our bodies by reducing inflammation, improving skin tone and strengthening joints. Supplement with omega 3 fatty acids and omega 6, and because not every fish oil is made the same please get the best your money can buy.

Probiotics

The wide spread use of antibiotics in the Western world means that much of our healthy intestinal gut flora has been reduced. Replenishing the 'good' bacteria is essential for fighting organisms that cause infections, so supplement with acidophilus containing acidbacilli and bifidobacteria.

So there you have it, a list of basic multi-vitamins and minerals that I use and that will support your body into a healing state. Most of the vitamins and supplements I have described here can be bought easily online. It is important, as I stated earlier, that you make sure you purchase good quality vitamins, ensuring they are not full of fillers like chalk, talc or soy.

Consult with your doctor, chemist, or pharmacist if you are concerned in any way prior to taking any supplements, especially if you are concerned that they might interfere with any current medications.

Ideally it would be best to have a doctor to support you in your desire to heal yourself naturally. Ask him or her to work with you and indeed use you as a case study to help other women. If complications arise in any way, shape or form contact your doctor who can readily make changes. They can take a look at why you are experiencing a reaction, if any.

Always start slowly with any supplementation, taking one supplement at a time. This is important; your body has been through enough stress, especially women who have had surgery, which is a traumatic experience on the body. All women with endometriosis have had to endure prolonged, intense periods of pain and upset, and this can make your body incredibly sensitive to ingredients. Introduce supplements slowly to gauge your bodies response to them and make sure that you do not have any undiscovered allergic reactions to these supplements.

If you find a supplement is too strong in its capsule dose form, then open the capsule and split the dose up. I was so ill when I started taking tablets that I had to split many of the supplements in to four doses and then slowly increase dosage as my body could adjust. Remember the aim is to get you well, not to make you worse: so go slow. "Slow is fast".

Chapter 17 -

Natural Aromatase Inhibitors

* * *

If you always do, what you have always done, you will always get, what you've always gotten - Wendy Laidlaw Anderson

I f you find you have removed all environmental

toxins, changed over your personal products including creams, lotions and perfumes, swapped your household products, drinking protein power shakes, eating hormone free meats and cut out wheat, sugar and soy, supplementing with multi-vitamins and minerals, as well as supplementing with natural bio-identical progesterone cream and are still experiencing pain, then it may be time to look at another layer in the battle against estrogen dominance and endometriosis in the body.

As we have discussed, estrogen dominance is a hormonal imbalance of excess estrogen and low levels of progesterone caused by a combination of poor diet, nutritional deficiencies, dioxins, xenoestrogens and phytoestrogens. These factors cause estrogen levels to increase in the body and inhibit the liver's ability to breakdown and expel estrogen. If you are poorly nourished from your diet, and have high estrogen, chances are you may have high levels of the enzyme aromatase. Excess aromatase in the body means that the inflammation cycle of endometriosis will be perpetuated.

Excess estrogen can also affect both the adrenal and thyroid glands, which in turn can make estrogen dominance worse. This is where natural aromatase inhibitors might be considered as an additional way of supporting your body into balance.

What is Aromatase?

Aromatase is an enzyme involved in the production of estrogen that increases the conversion of testosterone to one of the three estrogens called Estradiol. Aromatase is located in estrogen-producing cells in the ovaries, adrenal glands, testicles, fat tissue and the brain.

Natural aromatase inhibitors prevent the aromatase enzyme, and in doing so, lowers the level of two of the estrogens: Estradiol and Estrone. You will not be surprised to hear that medical aromatase inhibitors, prescribed by doctors and consultants, have side effects. Natural aromatase inhibitors are available in supplement form, although one natural way to acquire aromatase is eating vegetables rich in indole-3-carbinole.

In addition to increasing my intake of organic kale, cauliflower and broccoli, here are some of the natural aromatase inhibitor supplements I used in my healing journey:

I3C

I3C stands for 'indole-3 carbinole', which is found naturally in vegetables like cabbage, cauliflower and broccoli. I3C is a precursor to Diindolylmethane (DIM). I3C is available is supplement form.

Diindolylmethane (DIM)

Diindolylmethane (DIM) is a compound derived from the digestion of indole-3-carbinole, found in cruciferous vegetables, such as, broccoli, brussels sprouts, cabbage and kale and available in supplement form. DIM is purported to produce changes in the metabolism of unhealthy excess estrogen like Estradiol, whilst increasing levels of healthy estrogens like Estriol.

Myomin

Myomin is a formula of Chinese herbs produced by Chi's Enterprises and contains natural ingredients aralia, smilax glabra, curcurma zedoria, and cyperus rotundus. These herbs have been traditionally been used for various female ailments and hormone related disorders. Clinical trials show Myomin helps metabolise unhealthy estrogens; Estradiol and Estrone, and metabolises them into the good form of Estriol. Myomin is natural aromatase inhibitor and helps support over-worked adrenal glands. Curcurma has also been found to have antioxidant, antiviral, anti-inflammatory and immune boosting effects.

Calcium D-Glucarate

If I3C, DIM and Myomin do not help you get the desired results you may want to firstly consider increasing the dosage and then adding Calcium D-Glucarate to your regimen. Calcium D-Glucarate helps to make sure that hormones are not reabsorbed into the blood stream, where they may be deposited in the cells and tissue, but expelled from the body.

The natural aromatase inhibitors were particularly helpful in the elimination of all of my adenomyosis symptoms. Encouragingly for me, within a few weeks of taking the tablets the dragging sensations, contractions, 'bearing down' heaviness and vagina pain disappeared.

Despite being told by the gynaecologist that my only alternative was to have my uterus cut out, I had successfully identified the sources of my troubles and I had proved the doctors wrong again.

Chapter 18 -

Systemic Enzyme Therapy

* * *

Twenty years from now, you will be more disappointed at the things you didn't do, than by the ones you did - Mark Twain

Enzymes are proteins that are required for every single chemical action that takes place in your body. All of your cells depend upon the enzymes from your organs, muscles, bones and tissues. Your immune system, digestive system, bloodstream, spleen, liver, kidneys and pancreas, as well as your ability to see, think, feel, and breathe, are all dependant on enzymes.

In the immune system 'macrophages' (the Greek name for "big eaters") produce a wide array of powerful chemical substances including enzymes. These enzymes are formed in response to infection, dead or damaged cells. The job of the macrophages enzymes is to remove any cellular debris or dead cells that are found where they should not. As we already know with the displacement of endometrial tissue in the abdomen, endometrial lesions, cysts and adhesions are what macrophages are designed to 'clean up', but in women with endometriosis they do not do their job well.

Serrapeptase

Systemic Enzyme Therapy has a long history of being used in Germany, central Europe, Japan, and Mexico since 1950's, and is still used there today. One enzyme called Serrapeptase was used during a double blind study by German researchers on 66 patients. They discovered that those receiving Serrapeptase had a 50% reduction in swelling compared to the others in the study.

Assist your body in 'eating up' adhesions, cysts, and endometrial debris through systemic enzyme therapy supplementation and by consuming Serrapeptase.
Serrapeptase is naturally occurring proteolytic enzyme that is produced by the silkworm. The primary task of this enzyme is to breakdown the wall of the silkworm's cocoon before it turns into a moth. Serrapeptase was originally found in the intestines of the silkworm and is now processed through a naturally fermentation process in a laboratory.

Serrapeptase can also 'digest' and dissolve blood clots, arterial plaque and inflamed dead tissue within the body, as well as reducing pain, redness and swelling. Systemic enzyme formulas are backed by decades of clinical research and are also used for joint inflammation, Alzheimer's, angina to multiple sclerosis, prostatitis and respiratory infections. Serrapeptase helps to dissolve the billions of dead cells in the body naturally without harming the living tissue.

Many times I visited and asked doctors and gynaecologists why this product was not used or prescribed in the UK. Serrapeptase is used routinely in other countries as it is so safe, so effective and importantly has no side effects, and is a great alternative to painkillers. It has had many official studies to substantiate its effectiveness and has been used for over 40 years by more than 100 million people all around the world.

With regards to the quantity of Serrapeptase to take: I started with capsules of 80,000 IU. I moved up to 250,000 IU once I felt confident my body was happy with them. However, as I always caution, and even though there are no known side effects, please do start with smaller doses first to check how your body responds to them. After a few days you should begin to slowly increase until you feel positive effects.

Nattokinase

Nattokinase is another natural enzyme supplement that speeds up the biochemical reactions in the body. Like Serrapeptase, Nattokinase has been scientifically proven to benefit cardiovascular, blood clots, varicose veins and improving circulatory systems. Nattokinase works by breaking down 'fibrins' which are the fibres of blood clots and adhesions, they then dispel it from the body. Recent studies of this powerful enzyme have shown its effectiveness in reducing fibroids and cysts in women. Natto is boiled soybeans that have been fermented with a bacterium called Bacillus Natto. I was apprehensive about trying this supplement when I heard that it was made from soybeans. I contacted a few suppliers directly and I was reassured many times that although it is made from soy beans, the process of making Nattokinase actually takes the estrogen component out it.

Digestive Enzymes

Our body produces digestive enzymes are primarily created in the pancreas and small intestine. These enzymes help our body breakdown food so it can be absorbed in the intestines. When your body has had prolonged periods of time on pain killers, drugs, and surgery, or been under long periods of stress which inhibit natural enzyme production, the digestive process needs to be restored to a healthy balance. You will know if you need to supplement with digestive enzymes if you have any of the following symptoms;

> - undigested food in your stool
> - bloating after meals, gas or flatulence
> - hard sensation in your stomach

Unfortunately our cooked or processed foods destroy any enzymes that were naturally in the food, so you can see again why it is important to eat raw and freshly made food, or supplement if required.

Systemic Enzyme Therapy was the final piece of my endometriosis body puzzle. It took a few weeks to introduce them and I slowly built up the tablets to the point where I was taking Serrapeptase, Nattokinase, and digestive enzymes two to three times a day.

In addition to continued reduction in pain, I also noticed positive changes in other areas of my body including; regularity of my bowel movements (I had always suffered from terrible constipation), my nails got thicker, and the small surface cysts (on my ankle and on my nose) disappeared.

Finally, as with all other supplements, make sure that you read the ingredients list thoroughly. You would be surprised what some unscrupulous manufacturers pop into their capsules. You get what you pay for, so go for the best you can afford. I recommend capsules over tablets as they are easier to digest. How long you need to supplement for will depend on each person but for me it was for 3 months.

Chapter 19 -

Herbal Medicine

* * *

In the middle of difficulty lies opportunity - Albert Einstein

L et us begin to discuss herbal medicines. Herbal medicines are usually prepared by using the roots, flowers, stems, leaves, or barks of known medicinal plants. These preparations can be inhaled, applied as a topical salve, inserted as a suppository, or ingested orally in a tablet form or, as a drink (like tea). Often, different kinds of herbs are combined together to increase the effects.

One helpful effect from herbal medicine for endometriosis sufferers is the impact it can have on reducing excess levels of estrogen in the body. We already know that the liver is the main organ that can break down estrogen; herbalists suggest that the herbal medicine to be prepared should target the welfare and health of the liver. The most notable herbal preparation that is known to stimulate liver function is the combination of dandelion, beet leaves, cascara and uva ursi. The effect is not immediate; however, give it a few months of regular intake and one will feel free of symptomatic pain.

Various other herbs that are helpful in relieving endometriosis and symptomatic pain include; Cranberry, Plantain, Blue Cohosh, St. John's Wort, Peppermint, Valerian, False

Unicorn, Dong Quai, Evening Primrose Oil, Chasteberry, Black Cohosh, Uva Ursi, Couchgrass, Red Raspberry, Yam, and White Willow.

Chinese Herbs

In China, the treatment of endometriosis through the use of Chinese Herbal Medicine (CHM) is routine. There has been considerable research conducted into the role of Chinese Herbal Medicine and its role to alleviating pain, promoting fertility, and preventing relapse. Some studies claim that oral Chinese Herbal Medicine may provide a better overall treatment for relieving painful menstruation and shrinking cysts or lumps when used in conjunction with a Chinese Herbal Medicine enema.

Keishi-Bukuryo-Gan (KBG) - is a traditional Chinese herbal remedy and has been an approved prescription medication since 1970's. Keishi-bukuryo-gan has been used for the treatment of gynaecological disorders, such as hypermenorrhea, dysmenorrhea, and infertility. It is also very popular in Japan where some 40 million prescriptions are handed out each year.

Shakuyaku-Kanzo-Tos (SKT) - is a herbal formula traditionally used in Japan, Korea, and China. Studies have shown it reduces cysts and it is known to relieve menstrual pain, muscle spasm, and muscle pain.

Other helpful herbs

Vitex Agnus Castus - is popular in Europe for relieving menstrual difficulties and increasing natural progesterone production.

Chrysin - is a naturally occurring flavonoid in the chamomile, passion flowers, honeycombs, and certain mushrooms. It is a natural estrogen aromatase blocker stopping testosterone from converting into estrogen.

Cramp Bark - is a natural herb that helps to ease uterine cramps during menstruation.

French Maritime Pine Bark (also known as Pycnogenol) - is a powerful antioxidant which can also help with metabolising of excess estrogen and restoring hair loss.

Milk Thistle (Silybum Marianum) – is a wonderful herb that can help with liver detoxification. If I ever indulge in a glass of alcohol, I take two tablets prior to drinking and then, I take two more before I go to bed with a glass of water.

Asparagus Extract - this is a good herb at helping your kidneys detoxify. Symptoms of kidney issues can be lower backache, pain, and stiffness.

As with all medications, drugs, supplements or herbs, please do your own research before consuming them and consult your doctor if you have any reactions.

Chapter 20 -

Endometriosis Alternatives and Other Complementary Therapy

* * *

The quality of a person's life is in direct proportion to their commitment to excellence, regardless of their chosen field of endeavour
- Vince Lambardi

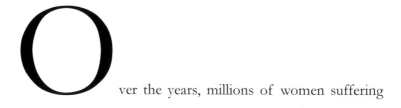

ver the years, millions of women suffering

from endometriosis have sought relief of their symptoms. Tired and fed up with the conventional medical approach, some of them tried to follow the complementary therapy way. These therapies may include any healing method from the use of herbs to varied pain management techniques. Many suffering women adopt them in an attempt to alleviate, or otherwise, manage a number of symptoms non-invasively.

Acupuncture
This ancient and traditional Chinese medicine involves fine needles inserted at certain sites in the body for therapeutic or preventive purposes. This is based on the belief that an energy, or life force, flows through our body via channels called meridians. Practitioners of acupuncture who adhere to this belief, believe that when this life force does not flow freely through our body, this will cause illness. The insertion of the fine needles is believed to restore the flow of this life force and thus restore health.

Acupuncture has been around for centuries and is still being applied today to treat pain conditions such as headaches, lower back pains, and osteoarthritis. It has also been reported to help people with conditions ranging from infertility, to anxiety and asthma. There are also some reports that acupuncture works for other problems, such as, neck pain and post-chemotherapy nausea and vomiting.

Acupuncture relieves general pain and is said to bring relief to women suffering from endometriosis pain, menstrual cramping, and even, post-operative pain. Unfortunately acupuncture is not readily available worldwide. There are even countries that outlaw it.

Myofascial Massage

Myofascial release massage is a specialised physical treatment for releasing tensions and restrictions caused by adhesions in the pelvic area. 'Myo' means muscle and 'fascia' means band. Fascia is connective tissue made of elastin and collagen fibres, surrounded by a viscous fluid. These two fibre types allow it to be very strong, yet have a high degree of flexibility and can respond well to manipulation through abdominal massage. Women with endometriosis can suffer from many adhesions that form due to inflammation and/or after surgery. Myofascial massage is an excellent natural alternative to having another operation to remove adhesions that may be wrapped around your internal organs. Another surgery may cause more adhesions and so the endless cycle would continue.

Myofascial massage was wonderful for me in helping break down my abdominal adhesions. The massage focuses on the abdomen area and is a very safe and effective technique, which releases the tightness of any fixed or tight adhesions into moveable and elastic fibres. After my 6th surgery I was in terrible pain and tightness in my abdomen. The myofascial masseuse was aghast when I turned up at her door, as I was hunched over looking like an 80 year old woman, unable to stand up straight. The treatment involves the therapist lifting and turning the abdominal skin and manipulating the layers underneath. It sounds sore but it was merely a little uncomfortable at times. The treatment was worth the minimal discomfort so that I was able to stand up straight and have less pain. It took about 12 massage sessions before I started to feel more flexibility and fluidity in my abdomen.

TENS Electrotherapy

Transcutaneous Electrical Nerve Stimulation, or TENS, is the most commonly used electrical stimulation device to apply electrotherapy to the body for the treatment of pain. It has electrodes that can be placed over the area of pain or over the nerve supplying the area of pain. The user then can adjust the desired intensity of electrical stimulation and select either high or low frequency. The exact mechanism of electrical stimulation's beneficial effects is not known. However, it is thought that TENS may effectively treat pain by blocking the transmission of pain signals along the nerves. It also shows that electrical stimulation promotes the release of endorphin hormones, which are natural painkillers produced by our body.

Shiatsu

Shiatsu, which is also known as acupressure, is a Japanese finger-pressure technique that is similar to massage. With the same purpose as acupuncture, shiatsu is designed to help regulate the flow of energy within the body. This type of massage helps produce deep relaxation and increased energy levels. Apart from relaxation, shiatsu also has other benefits, such as; preventing skin wrinkling, relieving rheumatoid arthritis and muscle pain, relieving migraine headaches, easing women from menstrual cramps, aiding women in labour or helping babies turn in the womb and improving the circulatory and digestive system.

Relaxation and Mindfulness Meditation

Mindfulness meditation is used all over the world and is scientifically proven to have many health benefits. Mindfulness meditation therapy can manage pain and reduce stress, and the great thing about it is anyone can do it. Mindfulness meditation therapy is a very natural and safe way to treat and heal yourself.

When mindfulness meditation was first suggested to me, I thought I might have to sit cross-legged on top of a hill, making a 'humming' sound. It felt a slightly preposterous practice to do. I have to share that this type of meditation has been hugely beneficial to me, and when I have had a session, I equate it to feeling like l have been recharged after being plugged into an electrical socket.

To do mindfulness meditation, the first thing to do is change the brainwave into a relaxing and resting state, referred to as theta. Once you are able to slow down your brain rhythm this way, your heart rate, metabolism, breathing rate, and blood pressure lowers too. This theta state can be achieved quite easily by simply focusing on your breath i.e. breathing in for 7 seconds, holding for 4, and then gently pushing out your breath slowly for 11 seconds. Natural painkillers in your body called Endorphins, are released into your system leaving you in a peaceful state of mind, observing your surroundings without forming judgments or thinking about anything else.

Mindfulness meditating may need some practice especially if you are not used to doing it. You may find that thoughts are rushing in: like a jumpy chirpy chimp! However, after a while, you should find that you can clear your mind of thoughts and induce a comfortable deeper relaxed state.

Mindfulness meditation therapy is widely practiced nowadays, even in the offices of Wall Street. It can relieve nervous system problems such as headaches, anxiety, stroke, depression, epilepsy, and multiple sclerosis. For women who suffer from excruciating endometriosis pain, meditation therapy has been proven to help improve the immune system. It can also help when there are periods of stress or anxiety to 'just notice' the thoughts like clouds in the sky passing you by.

Another great thing about mindfulness meditation therapy is that it has no negative effects, only good ones. You do not need to spend any money because it is totally free. As a beginner, all you need is a little place of peace and quiet to start practicing calming down your active conscious mind. Try the many different Apps for guided meditations available on iTunes, many that are free, which encourage you lie back, enjoy and relax.

Do not worry about 'doing it right'; there is no right or wrong way. If you fall asleep, do not worry, as it is better for you and your body because you fall into a deeper relaxed state of sleep. Little by little, you will allow your mind and your body as a whole, to get into that slow, gentle rhythm and reach a relaxing state of calm. There is no better feeling in this world than the meditative level of calm and peace. When you attain that, you will ultimately learn to hear that little quiet voice within yourself and that can guide you in directions you need to take, along with this book, to be finally, victoriously free from endometriosis.

Thought Field Therapy (TFT) and Emotional Freedom Technique (EFT)

Thought Field Therapy was created by the psychotherapist Dr Robert Callaghan, when a patient of his had a water phobia, which after many years, could not be cured. Quite by accident, after reading about the meridian systems used in acupuncture, Dr Callaghan discovered that if you 'tapped' on the acupuncture point with your fingers, then, stagnant energy would move, and along with it, the negative thoughts or anxious feelings. I have to admit to being a little cynical and resistant to the idea of Thought Field Therapy and Emotional Freedom Technique when I first heard about them. However, I admit now that I am a complete convert. It is a very simple process but very effective. There are lots of videos on YouTube showing you how to do it - why not give it a try?

Exercise

Exercise can be a stress reliever and also a good depression fighter; this is because it improves peoples moods by stimulating various brain chemicals that will leave people feeling happier and more relaxed. However, exercise for many women with endometriosis is a point of controversy. It is hard to exercise when your body is wracked with pain, bloating and tenderness. Many women feel guilty or push through the pain and exercise anyway. I recommend all gentle types of exercise like walking and swimming over running, weights or going to the gym. When you start to heal and are out of pain consider trying yoga and pilates which are gentle forms of exercise that work at strengthening muscles without causing hard impact on your already, tender body. Even going to sit outside in the garden or in a park for 20 minutes a day has beneficial effects for the body and mind. Sitting out in the sun helps to naturally improve your vitamin D levels. The most important thing to remember is to go slowly and gently. After all, endometriosis is a workout on its own.

Stress Management

Stress can add a lot of pressure to your already pained body so whenever possible make time for yourself to rest in a deep healing way. through relaxation exercises, breathing exercises or mindful meditation as mentioned earlier. This might be a challenge to start with. When stress management was first suggested to me I became aware of just how difficult it was for me to 'destress', as I was always in this mind set that I was somehow lazy or there were loads of things needing done. Even when I was so ill I could barely sit up or walk I knew I had to take decisive steps to get my body into a relaxed and healing state. This was hard work for me initially but persistency and consistency paid off. After a period of time and making an effort to allocate time to restorative rest, I started to notice a difference in my body. I was being less reactive to every day stressors and being more present in the moment.

Stress can come from many sources; work, relationships, financial and in the case of endometriosis, prolonged pain, and lack of information. Other stress factors might be caused by not feeling in a safe environment or living with an aggressive partner or workmate. When your body is in a constant state of stress your nervous system can get stuck in the 'flight or fight' response, sometimes referred to as a maladaptive state. The 'flight or fight' response is essential when you are faced with a sabre toothed tiger in your midst and is designed to protect you from danger. However, as mentioned earlier, to remain in this high vigilant state for long periods can actually add more stress and perpetuate any problems in your body. For example, the digestive tract stops functioning. Food consumed may not be broken down properly causing irritation and inflammation like irritable bowel syndrome (IBS).

Turn off your mobile phone, unplug your house phone and create a sign for your bedroom door saying "Relaxation in Progress: DO NOT DISTURB" and take some essential 'Me Time'. That was what I had to do for myself to carve out the essential escape from people and situations that were demanding my attention. I was so good at being there for other people but could barely look after myself. It is time to dedicate to yourself because you are worth it (as the L'Oreal advert says). Your body requires you rest it regularly so it can get a chance to heal. I suggest that a minimum of 20 minutes a day (or more) be allocated to trying some or all of the techniques. I hope you find the above as restorative as I have done.

Wendy K Laidlaw

Chapter 21 -

The 12 Basic Principles

* * *

The difference between the impossible and the possible lies within the person's determination - Tommy Lasorda

L ike any new routine, it may be challenging to

start with. It is said that it takes 21 days to form a new habit, so you should expect that applying the new ideas and the 12 basic principles of healing endometriosis naturally to take at least that period of time. It may take longer to form a routine depending on your level of commitment and economic resources. Healing endometriosis naturally is no 'quick fix' remember, but a permanent life style change.

It took me about 16 weeks to see and feel a difference. Some people achieve relief quicker, for others, it takes a bit longer. The key is to never give up. The principles take time to implement. Sometimes, it can be a mental adjustment of belief systems, as we are reluctant to 'give up' a food or product that is making us ill. There may be some questioning of beliefs about who is responsible for your body. Ultimately, we are responsible for our own bodies as we are the ones that have to live in them after doctors have finished 'tinkering' with them. You may want to stop and ask yourself, if the body is always wanting to heal itself, then what is stopping it and put on your detective hat.

It's time to let go of what is holding you back, reclaim your own power and follow your instincts to get out of pain.

Get on the healing path, get well and get out of pain.

These new habits will be the difference to you remaining in pain, with a hot water bottle attached to your abdomen for the rest of your life, or breaking free and moving forward. The aim is to get you living the life you deserve to live; pain free and fulfilling the destiny you were sent here to fulfil. Endometriosis sufferers deserve to be able to actually enjoy their lives before their time here passes. Some many women with endometriosis have spent lives just surviving; the time to thrive is up ahead. Just take the first small step, then the next.

The level of pain and symptoms in your body will depend on the level of changes that you need to make in your life. For results to be seen, changes will need to be made. Do not expect health to magically 'rain down' upon you.

To see results, you need to take _ACTION_

When you commit to these routines, you will reap the benefits. These new routines changed my life. Yes, I had to make changes. Yes, it was hard at times. BUT I am loving being pain free and having no pelvic pain or endometriosis symptoms. It is worth the changes I made and the bumps in the road I had to have got where I am now. It took me 14 years of extensive research and experimentation to learn the principles in this book. Now you have all that I learned in your hands to take control of your body and your life.

Expect that you may get a little frustrated or despondent, and you may even 'fall off the wagon' at times. Like falling off a horse or a bike, just get back on, (without beating yourself up) and keep on going.

I encourage you to set yourself realistic goals and also to have the odd 'treat'. When you have your 'treat', allow yourself one of your favourite foods as a treat for yourself; it can be anything from a chocolate bar or packet of crisps (making sure they have NO wheat in them though). Assuming you have achieved your intermediate goals, whether it be something like replacing your toxic washing powder with non-toxic organic coconut based washing powder for example, then have a 'treat' to reward without guilt. Never deny yourself any type of food as you may find you crave it more. Just negotiate with yourself, set a goal, achieve it and then treat yourself. This philosophy has worked wonders for me and my children. Then, after you have had the treat(s), notice how your body feels after eating it and then, get back on the wagon. Remember, you want to leave the pain behind, so re-commit to yourself, and keep recommitting to yourself, to getting back on the path to healing and to a pain free body.

Like going through the layers of an onion, the principles of Heal Endometriosis Naturally book is about helping you to identify which of the many sources are increasing inflammation and pain. Expect to become quite adapt at establishing, discovering and unfolding what the sources are that are causing you pain. It is time to take back control and responsibility of your body, and your life.

Here are the 12 basic principles below:

1) Test for hormonal, nutritional, and stomach imbalances

If you have the financial resources to do consider getting a saliva test done for estradiol, progesterone, and cortisol, along with a hair analysis test for nutritional deficiencies. Ask your doctor to test for B12 and ferritin iron blood levels. Consider doing the home test for stomach acid using the bicarbonate of soda test and getting a hair analysis test done.

2) Avoid All Wheat Products

If you only try one thing from this book make sure you try cutting out wheat flour from your diet for a minimum period of 3 months. Did you know that 83% of women with endometriosis also have a wheat intolerance, rather than issues with gluten? Look for items containing possible hidden wheat on the label that may say; dextrin's, modified starch, maltodextrin's, MSG-monosodium glutamate, malt, wheat germ flour, spelt flour, wheat germ oil, wheat pectin, wheat glucose syrup, thickening, couscous, semolina, cereal filler, rusk, bran, soy sauce, lagers, and beers.

3) You Are What You Eat

Eating healthy, fresh, free range, organic fruit and vegetables plus grass fed, hormone free meat, poultry, and fish, is essential and more details about diet will follow. Try goat's milk or coconut milk as an alternative to cow's milk. Fresh line caught fish but not from a fish farm: frozen fish from the supermarket is inexpensive, easy to store in bulk and super easy to cook. My favourite meal is cooking defrosted fish in coconut oil with some garlic and herbs; it is really delicious. Nuts and seeds are excellent sources of protein as are beans and pulses. Some women do well to exclude dairy from their diet whilst others are ok consuming it. Take your time to establish if your body is having a reaction to any foods by keeping a food diary. Keep a record of what you eat and how you feel, along with any physical reactions after you have eaten it.

4) Stomach Acid Test

Remember to test to see if you have enough hydrochloric acid in your stomach by doing the simple home bicarbonate of soda test. Take good quality digestive enzymes with every meal. You can eat all the good food in the world but if you are unable to breakdown and digest the food it will all be in vain. Fully absorbing and the elimination of waste regularly will be covered in later chapters too. To replenish your 'good' bacteria in your bowel you may want to also consider taking an acidophilus supplement. Nutrients from your food are absorbed in your small bowel through the lining into your blood stream. However, if the body is in a constant state of stress (in 'fight or fight' mode) the digestive tract stops functioning. Food consumed may not be broken down properly as digestive juices produced in the stomach called, hydrochloric acid, may not be present to do so. This means that undigested, unbroken down pieces of food may enter the intestinal track causing irritation and inflammation like irritable bowel syndrome (IBS).

5) Increase Protein Intake

If pain has dampened your appetite and you are struggling to eat solid foods, it is essential that you 'drink' your daily nutrients and calories. If you are not consuming at least 1,500-2,000 calories a day you will feel weak and struggle to do even the basic tasks. Your organs require nutrition and fuel to carry out even the basic bodily functions. Remember that it is bet to avoid synthetic products like Quorn as it is an edible fungus and tofu which is made from soybeans.

Increase your protein consumption to a minimum of 30 grams a day and aim to have a protein shake every morning. Within one hour of waking make a protein shake consisting of a pint of water/juice or coconut milk, two tablespoons of rice or pea organic protein powder (make sure it is not genetically modified i.e. Non-GM), crush two good quality multi vitamin and mineral tablets (like Solgar) or use rice based multi-vitamin and mineral powder, and 'Macro Greens'. One teaspoonful of Macro Greens is the equivalent of five fruit and vegetables a day. You may also want to invest in a juicer to start juicing your organic vegetables and fruits.

6) Correct Nutritional Deficiencies

Take a good quality multi-vitamin and mineral every day. Heavy, prolonged bleeding and blood clots can make a lot of endometriosis woman deficient in iron. Ask your doctor to check your ferritin iron levels and dependant on the results correct nutritional imbalances.

7) Remove Toxins and Estrogen Mimickers

Swap all plastics for ceramic and glassware. Stop cooking food in plastic and using the microwave, and get cooking in the oven using ceramic. Swap out hair, make-up, personal and household products that contain chemicals, parabens or SLS's. Swap chemical laden washing powders for coconut-based products instead, but again check the labels for any unwanted chemicals. Be aware that nail varnish and hair dyes are particularly toxic. Peel all non-organic fruit and vegetables. Cease the use of all synthetic and chemical drugs including painkillers if possible.

8) Natural Progesterone Cream

Consider getting a saliva hormone test done for progesterone and estradiol. Supplement with natural bio-identical progesterone cream to correct progesterone deficiencies and hormonal imbalances. Check over ingredients as you are looking for paraben and SLS free; and go organic if possible.

9) Natural Aromatase Inhibitors

Support your body's natural healing mechanisms to metabolise excess estrogens using supplements like natural aromatase inhibitors like DIM, Myomin, Pycnogenol or I3C.

10) Systemic Enzyme Therapy

Use natural enzyme supplements such as the well studied Serrapeptase or Nattokinase that have anti-inflammatory effects and can help dissolve, reduce and prevent blood clots, adhesions, and cysts. Use digestive enzymes with every meal to ensure you get the maximum nutritional benefit from your food.

11) Befriend Your Body

You are beginning a journey of learning about yourself and befriending your body. You will learn how to listen to your body, and how to interpret the signs and messages it is giving you. Up until now, your body may have just been this 'vessel' to carry your head around. You may have even hated your body for causing you so much pain and distress. Start by just noticing the people in your life who are energy draining, energy neutral or energy giving. You might be surprised at what you notice - but don't feel guilty, whatever the discovery is, even if it is a family member or close friend, just make a point of noticing it. Listen to your 'gut' instincts as your body is always trying to communicate with you. Listening to your body will become very empowering for you as you progress through the principles. The strengthening of this relationship with your body will be a focus during these next few months.

12) Journalling

As you are recovering from endometriosis you may start to re-examine some areas of your life. An excellent way to increase your awareness of what works and what does not work for you is to write a journal or diary entry every day. In Julia Cameron's book, 'The Artist Way', she refers to this journaling process as ' The Morning Pages'. It is a way to record your thoughts, feelings, self-pity, anxieties, fears, and hopes; really, whatever comes to mind. There is no wrong way to write your journal, but I would recommend you do it for at least a period of 12 weeks. Every morning upon wakening, take 20-30 minutes to write down the first things that come to mind on 3 sides x A5 page; don't worry if all your write is "I don't know what to write!" Some mornings even though I had not even slept, I wrote anyway. I wrote when I was sad, depressed, anxious or just plain puffed out with it all. I wrote even when all I felt was just plain negative. However, you might be surprised how you feel AFTER you have written out all that is going on in your head. A word of caution though: keep these words private to you for now.

This is about you and only you. You are writing a diary to record your progress, hear your inner voice, and monitor reductions in pain and/or symptoms.

If writing on paper does not feel safe or private enough, then there are some great journalling Apps online. Journaling was and still is a great way for me to see and mark my progress. I understand that you may think you will never forget this period in your life; all the pain and suffering you are enduring, but you will - because I did! It was only when I went back and reread my old diaries did I realise the progress I had made and just how much pain I was in - but also just how wonderful it is to be out of pain now.

Journalling is a great way to hear your dreams for the future and what is within your heart and soul. That little voice has been drowned out by pain, perpetual worry, busyness, thinking about others, and background anxiety; now is the time to think about yourself and your future.

Chapter 22 -

Begin your Healing Journey

* * *

Don't be afraid to take a big step if one is indicated; you can't cross a chasm in two small jumps - David Lloyd George

From all of this flood of information, I can safely say that all who suffer from endometriosis should treat it like a fire. Fire stays alive for as long as there is something to burn and oxygen to breathe. Take away any one of those two elements and fire will just go out. In the same fashion, we should also take away the various elements that endometriosis feeds on. By doing so, we are depriving it of its source of life and eventually it will just die out. Just like fire.

Now, we know that endometriosis is caused by the abnormal growth of endometrial tissue outside of the uterus, instead of lining the inside where it normally should. Medical experts have not fully determined why this happens and what causes the tissue to travel outside of its natural environment.

The principles behind Heal Endometriosis Naturally are to address endometriosis at a cellular, deep root level. Conventional medicine misses several stages of the endometriosis and tries to manage the symptoms rather than identify and eliminate the underlying causes. Medical treatment does not heal endometriosis. Painkillers, drugs and surgery routes merely keep you in an endless deteriorating cycle of chronic debilitating pain, hormonal changes, enzyme disruption and organ malfunctions. The Heal Endometriosis Naturally process stops infertility, eliminates pain, restores energy and amends the damage that has been caused to your body by the medical process.

We know that endometriosis is an estrogen dominant condition. A condition where a woman's body must maintain progesterone and estrogen at a normal ratio of 30 to 1. Therefore, how do we avoid this hormone imbalance? Obviously, we need to prevent the estrogen levels from going up. The very first step to do is to be very mindful of our environment. As we have discussed in earlier chapters estrogen can be found on just about anything from plastics, to cosmetics, to food, and many more. Check all of the things that you have around the house. Take a close look at the ingredients in your cosmetics, toilet-cleaning agents, dairy and food products. If there are ingredients that are alien to you or if you cannot pronounce their names, chances are these can be harmful to you, and worse, may contain estrogen mimickers. Discard these things right away, if finances allow, to avoid further contamination. Package up all of the offending items in a box and donate them to a charity or a friend. If you cannot afford to replace them immediately, then as you they out replace them; but research the alternatives in advance.

I have mentioned that estrogen is also present in the food that we eat. This hormone is mostly found in processed food, from vegetable and grain farms heavily sprayed with pesticides, and from livestock heavily induced with growth hormones. Therefore, when you go out to shop for food, be sure to buy only the freshest fruits, vegetables, fish, and meat. For the meat, try to investigate if the source is wild, free range, hormone free, and grass fed. In the UK there are many online companies that provide wonderful unprocessed, organic, hormone free food and will deliver direct to your door. Many at surprisingly low prices too.

If you decide enough is enough and you are going to commit to getting yourself out of pain, then from this point on you need to discipline yourself to have the patience to prepare your food. If you are a busy person and your work demands a lot of your time during the day, then you need to devise a time management plan to include food preparation in your daily schedule. Make time to think ahead. This is where I fell down initially and made it harder on myself, by not putting enough forward planning in. Because you are buying nothing but fresh food, these need to be prepared and cooked as soon as possible to avoid spoilage. Take advantage of online companies, who will deliver a box full of fresh organic ingredients, all ready to be prepared and made into a delicious and wholesome fresh meal.

Indulge yourself with protein rich diets. Remember if you are in so much pain and you are struggling to eat solid food, make your endometriosis protein power shake every morning and pour in all of that goodness to assist your body in its healing. Ample concentrations of protein in our body keep all of our vital internal organs healthy. Once we attain that proper and healthy balance of food intake, we make our liver happy. Moreover, if our liver is working properly, we will no longer worry about our estrogen levels going up.

We need to keep our bodies active but only if we are able. We should try and find time to engage in some small amount of physical activity, even if it is only a short walk or sitting outside for 20 minutes per day. When you are out of pain yoga, pilates or swimming are gentle and supportive ways to strengthen your body.

For some of us, the idea of making a change may seem like a daunting and arduous task. When we are in constant, chronic, and even, persistent low level pain, it can be hard to function on a daily basis, let alone think about what to eat, go out, purchase it and then cook it. If you are in a lot of pain with no appetite, I encourage you, at the very least, have one protein power shake every day, as previously mentioned. You will be amazed at how even that one small change can make a big difference.

You will now have to commit to making a complete lifestyle change. Go out and shop around for everything that is 'green', paraben free, SLS free, organic or made from natural ingredients. There are natural alternatives for cosmetics too. As for cleaning products, there are many do-it-yourself alternatives that use only natural ingredients. The internet is full of many wonderful suggestions.

Our body is not a separate entity from our minds and we are interconnected with our toxic environment and pollutants. Just like a rain drop is part of a weather system and a leaf part of a tree, endometriosis is part of the wider picture.

What we are looking to do here is to take small steps, and make one small change at a time.

Equally, it can be really tempting to go rushing in with great enthusiasm and want to do everything and change it immediately. Please don't do that either. All that will happen is you may get overwhelmed, confused and frustrated, then grind to an exhausting halt. You are in this for the next 12 weeks or so and hopefully beyond, so pace yourself for the long haul and give yourself realistic goals.

Many times, I zoomed down a path of treatment at 100 miles per hour like I was the old cartoon character 'Road Runner' on speed, bursting with enthusiasm, prepared to fully embrace my new find. Then after a short time I got stuck, hit a wall, burnt myself out and lost direction. This is where my motto 'Slow is Fast'. I learned to integrate the new principles and ideas slowly but most importantly, to bring back into

BALANCE all areas of my body and my life. My life was forever out of balance before, like my estrogen and progesterone levels, when I was in chronic pain. Balance is a very delicate thing and different for everyone.

I was in a very distressed and painful state five years ago and naturally, I, like most women, wished for a magic wand to come along and give me a 'quick fix' instantly. However, life does not work like that. I learnt that it had taken me a long time to get into the condition I was in and it was going to take quite some time to get the balance back into my body. I also learned that when I tried to rush the change it ended up taking me longer. Consistency and persistency is the key!

Every woman is unique and different, so each recovery journey will be personal to the individual woman. However, there are some commonalities and areas that we can assess to help us get started, on track and ultimately, to get you out of pain; naturally.

It takes time to see the results. When I get asked "Wendy, how long before I can start to see results?" my answer is always the same. What worked for me was a 50% reduction in pain within four weeks. Thus, continuing to follow the principles resulted in the total elimination of pain within 12 weeks. But everyone is different, so what works for one woman may not work for another. You have the 12 basic principles and roadmap now. Just keep on the road, apply the basic principles and never, ever, give up.

You will be becoming your own detective about your body, learning to listen and notice how your body is responding to the principles. You will learn to make adjustments or move to the next step when your body is ready.

But most importantly, be kind, compassionate and gentle on yourself; the pain of endometriosis has beaten you up enough...

And as Winston Churchill so eloquently said -

"Never, ever, ever, ever, ever, ever, ever, give up.
Never *give up.*

- Winston Churchill

Chapter 23

Support

* * *

Destiny is not a matter of chance; it is a matter of choice. It is not
something to be waited for but rather something to be achieved.
- William Jennings Bryan

Support is available in many forms if you get stuck or feel like you need a moral boost; but please, no matter what, do *NOT* ever give up hope. Join an online group or forum to reassure yourself you are not alone, ideally ones that supports a natural approach to healing.

Expect to be frustrated, impatient, and have the odd set back at times. That is normal. But, do not lose hope, get back on the path again, recommit to yourself and keep moving forward. Have faith that your body wants to heal itself and you have the power to do that.

If you hit a period of no progression, go back to step one and reread the information in this book. What have you missed or are missing? What has 'snuck' back into your diet, household products, personal products or routine that you had not realised? Are you taking adequate supplements, eating enough protein or had a hormone test done? Have you tried natural progesterone cream, the systemic enzyme therapy or natural aromatase inhibitors? Check what works for you, keep listening to your body and keep a record of your progress in your journal.

One day I would love to hear and read about your journey to a pain-free body and healing your endometriosis naturally. Your journey from surviving and struggling in pain, to thriving and hearing about your success. Then maybe working along with me to spread the word, and educate, empower and inspire other women to heal their endometriosis naturally.

If you need more one-on-one support and advice please contact me at Wendy@HealEndometriosisNaturally.com.

You are not alone and resources, webinars and trainings available online at WWW.HealEndometriosisNaturally.Com.

Sending you all of my healing love and hugs,

Wendy xx

Final Overview

∗ ∗ ∗

Opportunities are usually disguised as hard work, so most people don't recognise them - Ann Landers

Seven Steps & Basic Principles

Step 1	Nutritious Food & Protein Shakes
Step 2	Nutritional Supplementation
Step 3	Toxin & Xenoestrogen Removal
Step 4	Aromatase Therapy
Step 5	Hormone Therapy
Step 6	Systemic Enzyme Therapy
Step 7	Emotional & Brain Wise Therapy

No Wheat, No Wheat, No Wheat, No Wheat, *Absolutely* No Wheat

No Soy Or Soya

No Quorn

No Coffee

Stop - Iud/Coils

Stop - Birth Control Pill

Stop - Using Microwave

Stop - Using Plastic Containers & Kettle

Stop - Pharmaceuticals And Drugs

Stop - Pain Killers (If Possible)

Test - Hormone Tests

Test - Nutritional Deficiency/B12/Ferritin

Test - Digestion Betaine Stomach Acid Test

Test - Liver Function

Test - Stress Cortisol

Swap Out -   Toxic Personal Products

Swap Out -   Toxic Household Procucts

Swap Out -   Toxic Washing Powers

Eat -   30Gm Protein A Day Minimum

Eat -   Endometriosis Protein Power Shake

Eat -   Organic Free Range Food

Eat -   Cavewoman Diet

Introduce -   Nutritional Supplements

Introduce -   Natural Aromatase Inhibitors

Introduce -   Natural Bio-Identical Progesterone

Introduce -   Systemic Enzyme Therapy

Introduce -   Emotional Support

Identify -   Toxic People & Relationships

Identify -   People & Activities; Who Is -

Energy 'Giving', Energy 'Taking',

Energy 'Neutral'?

Start -   Mindfulness Meditation

Start -   Relaxation Exercises

Start -   Journalling & Daily Diary Writing

Try -   Yoga

Try -   Breathing Exercises

Wendy K Laidlaw

Meal Options

* * *

We are what we repeatedly do. Excellence then is not an act, but a habit - Aristotle

There are many wonderful wheat free and gluten free cook books out now but the main theme we are looking to follow is 'fresh is best'. Experiment with basic ingredients like free range organic eggs and become creative making omelettes or pancakes or even have a boiled egg. Eggs are very cost effective and full of nutrition. Below are some other ideas to get you started.

Breakfast Choices
Rice or other gluten-free cereal, with goats milk and blueberries or other fresh fruit.

Corn tortillas, warmed, with scrambled eggs, chopped tomato, and melted cheese.

Cream of rice with chopped almonds and coconut or goats milk.

Waffles with butter and agar syrup.

Omelettes with onions, peppers, and tomatoes.

Porridge Oats with fruit or agar or rice syrup.

Cottage cheese and fruit.

Homemade gluten & wheat-free flour pancakes with agar or rice syrup.

Dairy free yogurt (such as Coyo) layered with berries.

Ricotta cheese mixed and layered with berries.

Hard-boiled eggs mixed with mayonnaise, served on toasted gluten & wheat-free bread.

Bacon (Free range hormone free).

Sausages (Free range hormone free, wheat free).

Organic or frozen fruit.

Lunch Choices

Sliced turkey with lettuce, tomato, and mayonnaise on warmed corn tortillas with baby carrots.

Grilled sliced chicken over mixed greens, with red peppers, sliced tomato, broccoli florets, and chickpeas, served with oil and vinegar or wheat free salad dressing.

Toasted wheat free bread with tuna fish made with mayonnaise, chopped onion, sliced tomato, shredded lettuce, and chopped cucumber.

Grilled salmon or tuna served over mixed greens with shredded carrots, chopped tomatoes, and cucumbers. Serve with oil and vinegar, or favourite wheat free salad dressing, rice crackers, and lemon wedges.

Grilled chicken, salmon, or tuna, with shredded lettuce, sliced tomatoes, baby carrots, and rice cakes.

Gluten-free ham on wheat free toast with mustard and coleslaw.

Cottage cheese with mixed fruit.

Grilled chicken cutlet marinated in garlic, oil, and lemon, served over chopped romaine lettuce, with wheat free Caesar dressing, parmesan cheese, and rice crackers.

Grilled or broiled sirloin burger with lettuce, tomato, sliced onion, catsup, and a wheat free roll if available serve over a mixed salad with oil and wheat free vinegar.

Grilled chicken marinated in garlic, oregano, oil, salt, and pepper, with a sweet potato, butter, and mixed veggies.

Chicken salad made with cooked chicken, mayo, onions, walnuts, and grapes, over a mixed green salad.

Grilled mushroom marinated in garlic and oil, served with mixed green salad.

Dinner Choices
Salmon baked with mustard and honey, served with brown rice and steamed green beans.

Hardboiled egg, sliced, with steamed green beans, baby spinach,sliced cucumber, sliced tomato, and chickpeas with oil and vinegar or gluten-free salad dressing.

Grilled chicken cutlet marinated in garlic, oil, and onion powder, served with cooked brown rice, steamed broccoli, and mixed greens served with oil and vinegar or gluten-free salad dressing.

Cooked kidney beans and brown rice added to chopped onions sautéed in olive oil with garlic, and with chopped tomato, chopped red pepper, and hot pepper added to taste, served with a green salad and wheat free dressing.

Broiled skirt steak with garlic, onion powder, and a dash of salt, served with steamed cauliflower and a medium baked potato with butter.

Baked flounder cooked with chopped onions, tomatoes, cilantro, garlic, and onion powder, served with steamed spinach, rice, and a mixed green salad with sliced tomato and cucumber and oil and vinegar or wheat free salad dressing.

Pork loin cut into two-inch cubes and placed on a skewer with chunks of pineapple, cherry tomatoes marinated in wheat free dressing, grilled, and served with steamed broccoli and corn with butter or margarine and a dash of salt.

Roasted chicken with carrots, potatoes, and onions, seasoned with garlic, onion powder, salt, pepper, and Italian herbs.

Grilled or baked chicken, shrimp, or veal, placed in a casserole dish and topped with tomato sauce, mozzarella, and parmesan cheese, served with gluten-free pasta.

Brown rice, corn, or quinoa pasta with tomato sauce and a mixed green salad with favourite gluten-free dressing.

Grilled shrimp over a mixed salad with baby potatoes and favourite wheat free salad dressing.

Hand-pressed hamburger or turkey burger, with onion and sliced tomato, baked sweet potato fries, and green beans.

Frozen wheat free pizza baked and served with mixed green salad and wheat free salad dressing.

Snack Choices
Organic fruit, Canned fruit in its own juice, Dairy-free yogurt, (such as Coyo), Organic carrots with hummus, String cheese with dried fruit, Rice cakes, Oat cakes, Nuts, Dried fruit.

Ingredients to Avoid
Wheat, Atta, Kamut, Bulgur, Matzoh Meal, Couscous, Modified Wheat Starch, Dinkel (also known as spelt), Seitan, Durum Semolina, Einkorn Spelt, Emmer, Farina Triticale, Farro or Faro, Wheat Bran, Fu Wheat Flour, Graham Flour, Wheat Germ, Hydrolysed Wheat Protein, Wheat Starch.

Xenoestrogens

* * *

Do it now - Napoleon Hill

Guidelines to minimise your personal exposure to Xenoestrogens:
- Avoid all pesticides, herbicides, and fungicides.
- Choose organic, locally-grown and in-season foods.
- Peel non-organic fruits and vegetables.
- Buy hormone-free meats and dairy products to avoid hormones and pesticides.

Plastics:
- Reduce the use of plastics.
- Do not microwave food in plastic containers but use glass instead.
- Do not use plastic wrap/cling film to cover food for storing or microwaving.
- Use glass or ceramics whenever possible to store or cook food.
- Do not leave plastic containers or drinking water in the sun.
- Throw away a plastic water container if it has been heated up.

Household Products:
- Use chemical free, coconut based, biodegradable laundry and household cleaning products.
- Choose chlorine-free products and unbleached paper products (tampons, menstrual pads, toilet paper, paper towel, coffee filters).
- Use a Britax filter jug, chlorine filter on shower heads and filter drinking water

Health and Beauty Products:
- Avoid creams and cosmetics that have parabens, SLS and stearalkonium chloride.
- Reduce your exposure to nail polish and nail polish removers.
- Reduce use of perfumes and use naturally based fragrances, such as essential oils.

- Use chemical, paraben, SLS soaps and fluoride free toothpastes.
- Read the labels on condoms and diaphragm gels.

Some of the named chemicals that are xenoestrogens:
- Skincare products- 4-Methylbenzylidene camphor (4-MBC)
- Sunscreen lotions - Benzophenone
- Body and face creams - Parabens called methylparaben, ethylparaben, propylparaben and butylparaben which are commonly used as a preservative

Industrial products and plastics:
- Bisphenol A (monomer for polycarbonate plastic and epoxy resin; antioxidant in plasticizers)
- Phthalates (plasticizers)
- DEHP (plasticizer for PVC)
- Polybrominated biphenyl ethers (PBDEs) (flame retardants used in plastics, foams, building materials, electronics, furnishings, motor vehicles).
- Polychlorinated biphenyls (PCBs)

Food:
- Erythrosine / FD&C Red No. 3
- Phenosulfothiazine (a red dye)
- Butylated hydroxyanisole / BHA (food preservative)

Building supplies:
- Pentachlorophenol (general biocide and wood preservative)
- Polychlorinated biphenyls / PCBs (in electrical oils, lubricants, adhesives, paints)

Insecticides:
- Atrazine (weed killer)
- DDT (insecticide, banned)
- TCDD (2,3,7,8-Tetrachlorodibenzo-p-dioxin)
- Dichlorodiphenyldichloroethylene (one of the breakdown products of DDT)
- Dieldrin (insecticide)
- Endosulfan (insecticide)
- Heptachlor (insecticide)

- Lindane / hexachlorocyclohexane (insecticide, used to treat lice and scabies)
- Methoxychlor (insecticide)
- Fenthion
- Nonylphenol and derivatives (industrial surfactants; emulsifiers for emulsion polymerization; laboratory detergents; pesticides)

Drinks:
- Avoid carbonated or fizzy drinks
- Aspartame is a substance the body cannot break down and floats around the body
- Saccharin
- Sugar
- Coffee

Other:
- Propyl gallate
- Chlorine and chlorine by-products
- Ethinylestradiol (combined oral contraceptive pill)
- Metalloestrogens (a class of inorganic xenoestrogens)
- Alkylphenol (surfactant used in cleaning detergents

Phytoestrogens:
Phytoestrogens are the most studied of all the phytochemicals and are weaker than the natural estrogen hormones. Although not as potent as other forms of estrogen mimickers it is best to avoid them. Some phytoestrogens are;
- Soy
- Soya
- Wheat
- Coffee
- Pomegranates
- Dates

ABOUT THE AUTHOR

Wendy K Laidlaw lives in Edinburgh, Scotland with her two
children and chocolate labrador.
Wendy is a woman's health author, consultant, nutritional therapist,
psychotherapist and endometriosis advocate.

Wendy K Laidlaw

Heal Endometriosis Naturally

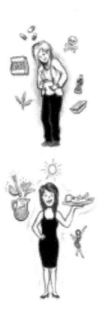

Wendy K Laidlaw